Disclaimer

The author and pu~~......~~   d the contents of this book to ensure that it is as accurate as possible at the time of publication.

The book is for information only, and has been researched in good faith and to the very best of our knowledge.

Please be advised that the information in these pages is not necessarily representative of the views of other health professionals or physicians. Do not treat it as a substitute for medical advice from qualified doctors or dieticians.

If you are pregnant, we advise that you seek professional advice before making any dietary – or other—changes to your lifestyle. If you have any concerns, however small, please seek medical attention before following any of the recommendations given in this book.

The Ultimate Guide to Antiaging – Look 10 Years Younger in 10 Weeks

Discover the Inside Story from an Ex-Nurse about Anti-aging Diet Strategies and Anti-Aging Tips for Skincare

Rosi Thomas

Contents

FORWARD

"You can't help getting older but you don't have to get old" George Burns

Hello and a warm welcome to "The Ultimate Guide to Antiaging", the little book with a big message that will change the way you think about your skin forever. Firstly I'd like to say "Congratulations" - you have taken that first all-important step towards achieving and maintaining beautiful, healthy skin **without** the price tag, **without** the pain (of costly time-consuming cosmetic treatments such as botox) and **without** any hidden "nasties" such as parabens which can dry or irritate the skin in the short or long-term.

You are going to discover simple skincare strategies that you can easily copy for sensational results every time - because they work! **Imagine it**...Looking in the mirror and seeing *a real and visible difference in your skin* - just knowing it's the best it can possibly be. **Imagine ...** the compliments you'll receive from family and friends, and how much more confident this will make you feel. **Imagine ...** having at your fingertips such powerful information and secrets that can slow down (and in some cases even reverse) the ageing process and promote a life-time of well-being.

To introduce myself, my name's Rosi, and I'm a retired nurse from The Midlands. I've always had a professional interest and insight into the fascinating subject of skin health/skin care, and how the skin is such a fantastic barometer by which to judge a person's overall health and lifestyle.

As you can imagine, I came across a whole kaleidoscope of skin conditions and complaints on the wards, from bed-sores and burns, to acne, eczema and psoriasis! I also became acutely aware of how adversely our skin reacts to certain factors such as illness, constant pain, poor diet or the ageing process – to name but a few. Personally however, as is often the case, it was an entirely different matter …

How well I remember working night shifts, all 22 years of them! Frequently stressed and exhausted, my body clock was all over the place due to lack of sleep. I was eating meals at all odd hours, constantly picking at biscuits and chocolates left to us by grateful patients – and smoking to deal with all of the above.

Having always been lucky enough to look younger than my age, and because after so many years this lifestyle was the norm for me, I had never really scrutinized myself in the mirror that closely – I think I must have imagined I was some sort of Peter Pan – and it was only after I turned 50, and in the aftermath of an unexpected hip replacement, that I suddenly became aware of what had been happening, slowly and insidiously, to my skin.

It was as if it had happened overnight. I remember one day noticing the back of my hands on the steering wheel, as if really seeing them for the first time. And there it was, the result of a lifetime of sun worship (using little, if any, protection), poor diet and poor lifestyle. Gone was the lovely smooth skin I had always been lucky enough to have, and in its place was an intricate web of small wrinkles which only disappeared if I clenched my wrists tightly.

To my horror, when I examined my hands even more closely, I also found one or two faint age spots developing.

This was a huge wake-up call for me, and for the first time I was forced to realize that I was actually getting – and, well, looking – older. Of course paranoia quickly set in! On inspecting my face and neck in the mirror at various angles (something I don't think I'd ever purposefully done before), I was horrified to find new, deep lines embedded in folds of skin at the sides of my mouth – and more than a hint of loose, saggy skin underneath my chin when I tilted my head or turned it from side to side. To top it all I discovered I had bunions (which I swear had arrived overnight) - not of course relevant to the subject of this book but nevertheless the final straw in a long list of afflictions!

How had this happened? How long had I looked like this? Had other people noticed what had been happening to my skin?? I had always been quite vain about my physical appearance, had always religiously cleansed, toned and used the newest and most expensive skin-care products I could afford. Plus, being a nurse, I understood all about the make-up and structure of the skin and the many conditions that can afflict it and had seen first hand how it can change like a barometer in response to both internal and external factors.

How could I have missed what was happening to my own skin, as a result of natural ageing added to years of what can only be termed abuse of my health, and despite having spent literally hundreds of pounds on expensive cleansers, toners and skin creams over the years? It was one of those weird situations where you see it happening to other people but never think it will happen to you. I very quickly realised that I needed to take myself in hand and clean up my act. The time had come when all the miracle creams in the world would not, on their own, correct the damage that had been wreaked from the inside. The truth was finally out.

Now however, several years later, having taken early retirement due to a back problem and having the time to think about myself and adopt a healthier lifestyle, I look and feel a different person - and it has become increasingly important to me to keep as young and healthy looking as possible.

As a result of my own experience, observations and research, plus a considerable amount of trial and error, I can now reveal the **ONE amazingly simple and natural solution** that keeps your skin radiant and glowing from top to toe (*yes, your whole body and not just your face*) and that also helps problem skin - a strategy that delivers sensational results every time BECAUSE it works! Anti-wrinkle creams?? Collagen creams?? Forget them! Been there, done that. There's a far better – and cheaper – alternative!

INTRODUCTION

"Beauty starts from the inside … and shines on the outside" Laura Tommons Quotes

The message at the heart of my book is this … that our skin is the mirror of our overall health, and the only way to keep your skin looking radiant, regenerated and relaxed is from the inside out - not from expensive anti-ageing creams which only temporarily mask the problems of ageing, rather like papering over the cracks in a wall.

This simple but powerful concept is one which many people hear but most don't want to believe. Reason being? Because they are brain-washed by clever advertising and the idea of little gold pots of expensive cream on their bathroom shelves which must work because the price tag says it will – and have subconsciously closed their minds to the possibility of a better, simpler and cheaper option that could actually work.

How many times in life do we ignore the glaringly obvious, believing that the answer we seek couldn't possibly be that simple? I've done it myself in the past, so I know! You only have to look at the number of adverts on your television screen, or in magazines or the national press, to realize that skincare is a multi-million pound industry - as is cosmetic surgery. These companies spend millions of pounds annually in advertising alone, to prey on the four most compelling emotions of women with regard to their looks:

DREAD : FEAR : VANITY : DESIRE

Dread

However much we try to pretend to the contrary, we all, for one reason or another, dread getting old. Some people are very much affected by the prospect from quite early on. I remember in my twenties, a friend saying she would rather die than get old, and this was a huge concern for her. Others develop an enviable gung-ho attitude towards life, embracing the fact that they have more freedom and no longer feel the need to prove themselves etc etc. But is this how they really feel? Or is it their (conscious or sub-conscious) way of coping with the inevitable?

We like to think that we are in control of most aspects of our lives, but one thing we will never be able to control is the passing of time and the fact that if we live long enough, and despite all our efforts to the contrary, we **will** eventually look our age. This may happen sooner, or considerably later, depending on many factors such as (very significantly) our genes, our mental attitude (namely how we see ourselves and what mentality we adopt) and how responsibly we look after ourselves throughout our lives.

Fear

Fear of physical ageing is responsible for all manner of things - people lying about their age, 20-30 year olds believing they are over the hill, and billions of dollars a year blown on Botox and cosmetic surgery. We fear wrinkles because of what we believe those wrinkles reveal about us, and because our physical appearance is important – after all it impacts on our innate confidence in ourselves, in the way we dress, in our activities, in our perception of how we are seen by family, friends, colleagues and the opposite sex. We are scared of looking in the mirror and seeing – as I did – wrinkled, saggy skin and new lines around our mouth and our eyes. It emphasizes the passing of time and causes us to consider our own mortality.

Vanity

The whole beauty industry is about pande helpless vanity and combating our fear of We smother our faces with lotions al containing all manner of "miracle" promising us youthful, radiant and regene even though some of these ingredient Retinol can have horribly adverse effects on some individuals.

The bravest and most daring of us go "under the knife" and are lifted, nipped and tucked by plastic surgeons in an attempt to defy gravity. We have breast reductions or insert implants to give us perkier looking breasts, and we have our foreheads and lips injected with botox and fillers when all the laser treatments and chemical peels fail to work to our satisfaction. Sometimes these procedures - as we see all too often in the press – have very nasty consequences indeed. So WHY do we do all this?

The answer of course is VANITY, the eternal quest for youth and beauty, the constant search for a magic remedy that will slow down the ageing process, even turn back the clock. But in so doing are we really aware of the risks we are taking with our health, or of what we're applying to our faces and our bodies? In some cases maybe so ... but vanity is a very strong emotion that will prevail over common sense, and it is for this reason that the beauty and cosmetic surgery industries continue to flourish and make their millions.

It is clear, from the increasing amount of horror stories we read in the press, that many companies offering cosmetic surgery and various procedures such as Botox are increasingly putting profit over ethics.

Desire

Clever advertising is all about "Desire". We see something, we want it - we may not *need* it but we *want* it, there is a not so subtle difference. Anyone who has seen the film "Out of Africa" starring Robert Redford and Meryl Streep, may remember Dennis Finch-Hatton's words to Karen in an intense exchange over their relationship: "You confuse need with want, you always have ...." How true this is of us women in general! **Why**, when barely halfway down our purchase of the latest miracle face cream, are we so compellingly hypnotized by the next new anti-ageing advertisement that appears to promise even better and quicker results than the product we bought only two weeks before? No, of course we do not need it, but because of clever wording and the compelling nature of the ad, we overwhelmingly DESIRE it, we are afraid of missing out, we HAVE to have it. Sound familiar?! I rest my case!!

The bottom line is this, that *it is pointless wasting your hard-earned cash on expensive lotions and potions to plaster on top of dull, lifeless or poorly nourished skin.*

If someone suffers from body odour and sprays themselves with expensive perfume, does it cure the problem? You know of course, that it does not, it merely masks it – and badly at that. If the bodywork on your car has a deep scratch, does it solve the problem simply to spray over the area and hope for the best? No, and worse still, *as you have now covered up the blemish, you are blind to the rot that continues to eat away at the bodywork beneath.*

There is a very real connection between diet and health and the appearance of your skin, and as your skin is on show to everybody it is very visible evidence of poor nutrition and other bad habits. You can't simply apply skin cream twice a day - however expensive and however many miracle claims it boasts – and expect long term results. It doesn't work like that. Whichever way you dress it up, all you are basically doing is re-hydrating the dead cells on your skin's surface - and this solution is, unfortunately, merely a temporary one.

Serious skincare begins and ends with your diet and lifestyle, period ... and I'm on a mission for you to realise that by using an internal health approach you can look up to 10 years younger in as little as ten weeks **if** you take action on the information you will find in this book.

WHAT YOU CAN EXPECT FROM THIS BOOK AND HOW BEST TO USE IT

"The path to success is to take massive, determined action." Anthony Robbins

Anybody of any age-group, male or female, should find the information in this book to be invaluable ... people with problem skin, young people looking to keep their youthful, natural looks for as long as possible, and older people looking to "turn back the clock" on ageing. For every single one of these individuals however, the core message is the same, that *to spend a fortune on external skincare is not only unnecessary but completely and utterly pointless.* The reasoning behind this will become clear to you as the book unfolds. In fact once you reach the end come back and re-read the following paragraphs again – it will all make absolute sense!

Section 1 is all about the HOW, WHY and WHEREFORE, the unadulterated facts about the structure and function of your skin from someone who has had 22 years experience in the medical industry, that will catapult your knowledge and understanding into the stratosphere! You will discover that you have not only one, but *three different ages*, and why this is so vital to your perception of the ageing process. You will also discover the truth about what wrinkles really are, and how and why they develop as part of a very natural and gradual process within the structure of your once flawless skin.

You will discover why these "15 deadly enemies" of your skin (there could be one or two you hadn't thought of) can accelerate your skin's natural ageing process by as much as 100%, and **why** your body's circulation is so fundamentally, vitally important to the whole anti-ageing issue.

Circulation is often given only very scanty consideration in books and articles relating to skin care, *a huge omission* as it is actually the root cause of all your health and beauty-related issues. It is **this** that you need to fully understand – to be shocked by even – before you are ready to take the simple steps that could "smash that clock" and knock at least 10 years off your biological age in as little as 10 weeks.

Everything you read in this book will ultimately trace back full circle to this one key issue. I strongly believe this to be a very different angle on the subject that will result in a higher level of understanding, not only of WHAT you need to do to turn back the clock on ageing (in itself not new information) but, in simply explained biological terms, precisely WHY you need to do it. Your success depends on you being able to see both sides of the coin. The ball is then in your court as to whether you take action to create a whole new head-turning "you" and to insure your skin for the future, or whether you do nothing. One thing is certain, if you do nothing then nothing will happen - except that the changes in your skin in years to come will almost certainly not be good ones.

You will probably need to read Section 1 several times before progressing to Section 2, but this is good as it shows you are serious and committed to making this work. You are fast becoming an expert, you are going to be able to educate and advise other people on this subject. *Read, learn and understand* - because only when you understand "*why*" are you ready to move on to "*how*". If what you read doesn't shock you into action then this book is probably not for you.

Section 2 is definitely information that the big skincare companies would prefer you didn't know: what lies behind their advertising campaigns and how you are conned into buying products that – for a very specific reason which I will go into later in detail – cannot possibly do what they claim: the truth behind cosmetic surgery and botox: the shocking substances that are blatantly added to the majority of trusted "brand-name" products you use every day and *why*, even though the manufacturers assure us they are in a small enough concentrations to pose no threat to health, it is the accumulated build-up over years of use that will eventually manifest itself in various health problems and rapidly ageing skin: and finally, why prolonged use of a moisturizer can actually cause your skin to become drier. Section 2 is definitely called "*The Myth, the Lies and the Truth*" for good reason.

Section 3: I have called Section 3 "The Plan" for want of anything more inspiring! However you will see that it is not a structured plan in the sense that a weight loss or exercise régime might be. Instead you will find a detailed yet simply explained analysis of certain facts of which you may not have been aware, and that will help you make important and informed decisions about your lifestyle. This is followed by a wealth of workable ideas and suggestions as to how you might best implement these decisions and incorporate the amazing benefits into your own personal and individual routine on a day-to-day basis.

One of the difficulties in writing this guide was the attempt to reconcile the amazing difference you can make to your skin - *if* you don't smoke, drink or eat any of the "bad" foods that can compromise your health and your looks – with what is sustainable for most of us in today's modern world.

The reality is that most of us, in part due to the busy lives we lead, are inherently lazy and are always looking for a "quick fix" – something that will do all the work for us and involve no effort on our part. This is the reason why most diets and fitness plans fail, started with such zeal and enthusiasm each new year only to fall by the wayside as the year gathers pace and "life" as always, takes over. It is the one thing that skincare companies rely on to explode the sales of their products, their clever marketing offering quick-fix "miracle" solutions in a jar to all those women *desperate* to keep their looks but without the time or inclination – and mostly without the knowledge - to do anything about it.

Well the honest truth is that there *is* no quick fix when it comes to your skin, which is a mirror image both of your current state of health and your past and present life-style. Problems in these areas are fundamental, and while – serious health problems aside – they can usually be addressed quite simply and with astounding results, this does involve a bit of thought and adjustment on your part.

For this reason I decided that to simply get down to the root of the matter in an honest, no-nonsense way that anyone, even with a non-medical background, can understand, would set the alarm bells ringing and even instill a healthy bit of fear! Because it is this fear - *"if you don't do* **this***, then* **this** *is what will happen"* - that will be the ultimate incentive you need to trigger you into action, and that I hope will nag away at you through all those times when your resolve is in danger of weakening! Read on for a small "taster" of some of the ideas you will find in this little book …

The plan I have set out at the end works very simply through *substitution* **of good habits for bad habits/good foods for bad foods**. I have tried to give emphasis to those things that you definitely should give up or at the very least, drastically cut down on - but to leave some leeway in other areas.

To a great extent it is about balancing the negatives against the positives, for example, weighing up the foods that contain no nutritional benefits whatsoever - the true "baddies" - against those that have a foot in each camp as it were, offsetting maybe only *one* bad point against some otherwise very valuable nutrients.

For instance, we now know that sugar is bad for us, and as honey contains around 3tsps of natural sugar per tablespoon, in theory it should be avoided. My own opinion however, is that a small drizzle of honey to sweeten an otherwise healthy dessert is a far better option than that rich chocolate brownie pudding with ice-cream, laden with *added and refined* sugar and fats, that you might previously have eaten - particularly if you opt for organic honey (with *Manuka* being the ultimate choice here) in order to take maximum advantage of all the *positive* health benefits that honey has to offer. For the small amount you will use it is worth spending more and making it last.

Treacle too, as you will see, actually contains *significant health benefits to offset its sugar content* – which means that if you want to indulge in the *occasional* spoonful then at least you are not just consuming empty calories.

And yes, there is natural sugar too, for example, in dried fruit - and added sugar (about 1tsps to every tbsp) in balsamic vinegar. However to eat a small handful of dried raisins or apricots as a delicious snack is so much healthier than biscuits, a chocolate bar or a bag of crisps, all of which are full of added and processed sugars, "bad" fats and "E" numbers, and with almost zero nutritional benefit to your skin.

A drizzle of quality balsamic vinegar (and as you will read later some brands now offer healthier alternatives with a lower sugar/salt content) to spice up a salad, is better than a bog-standard salad dressing high in sugar, fat and salt.

A slice of home-baked or organically produced fruit loaf is a far better option than a piece of pithy white bread, "off the shelf" and containing processed flour, sugar and salt with a dearth of other additives and preservatives (I hesitate even to call it bread). Are you beginning to get the picture?

So long as the balance is tipped weightily in favour of healthy, unprocessed ingredients, then a little bit of the other is ok if it means the difference between sticking with, or not, your newly reformed eating habits. And this is the reason why you might sometimes find the odd tablespoon of tomato ketchup or similar, lurking in the recipes at the end of this book!

Similarly, if you just love cake or steamed puddings, then to try to cut them out of your life altogether is, in my experience, a recipe for impending failure. It is unrealistic, and most people will not be able to keep this up indefinitely. So have one occasionally, but learn how, and/or put aside some time, to make your own - substituting healthy, unrefined ingredients for

18

past unhealthy ones and using a sugar alternative whenever possible.

Your cake or pudding won't taste any worse – in fact I promise you it will taste a whole lot better - for being made with an organic whole-grain flour, "whole" butter, and unrefined sugar (or sugar alternative), rather than with a processed flour that has been stripped of all its nutritional value, a low-fat margarine or cooking spread that is full of added sugar and chemicals, and a refined sugar that has zero health benefits and – to add insult to injury - will end up, like all sugar, being converted to fat in your body anyway (much more on this later).

Try to include at least one highly nutritious food in the recipe, such as fresh or dried fruit, some chopped or crushed nuts or some grated carrot or parsnip for natural sweetness, to offset the less nutritious ingredients. You will be surprised at how quickly this becomes a habit!

Almost any recipe can be adapted in this way, simply by substituting healthier ingredients for unhealthy ones. Home baking is only as bad as what you put into it, and if you stick to the rules there is no reason why, in sensible amounts, you should not enjoy the occasional "traditional pudding" or slice of cake.

The same principal of substitution applies when dealing with all those harmful factors that threaten your health and skin integrity on a daily basis. You may find it difficult to cut them all out of your life to begin with, but persevere, with small baby steps to begin with, because the reality is that every small change you make will accumulate over time to make a big difference, providing you maintain it.

The key is to gradually replace harmful products with non-harmful ones over a period of time. For example if you are trying to cut down on household cleaning products that contain alarming amounts of toxins and chemicals, yet find the prospect a daunting one, rather than feel under pressure to replace all your cleaning materials in one go - each time one of your current toilet cleaners, drain busters or pack of anti-bacterial wipes comes to an end, simply replace it with something more eco-friendly.

Once you are comfortable with one change, then work on making another and carry on doing this until you have successfully redefined your lifestyle (and your shopping list!). It may take you only two months, it may take you a year, but one thing is certain: if you put this simple plan into action then you will look and feel so amazing that you'll wish you had done it years ago!

Section One: Facing the Facts

Chapter One

In a nutshell: Eight things you may not know about your skin

Your skin is pretty amazing! It literally "holds everything together"! Did you know that …

1. It is the largest organ in your body with a surface area of around two square metres, and it makes up around 16% of your total body weight.
2. There are approximately six million cells per square centimeter of skin, all with various different functions.
3. It is made up of 70% water, 25% protein and 2% lipids. The remainder includes trace minerals, nucleic acids and numerous chemicals.
4. It contains nerve endings, blood and lymph vessels, hair follicles, cells for the production of melanin, and sebaceous glands.
5. It stores water, fat and vitamins and enables the synthesis of Vitamin D.
6. It is a natural barrier that protects your body from harmful substances, changes in order to regulate your body temperature, and allows you your sense of touch.
7. It is a mirror of what is going on within the rest of your body. Have you ever heard anyone described as having an "*inner beauty*" or an

"*inner glow*"? That is because your skin presents a first impression to the rest of the world. If it is radiant and glowing with the sort of beauty that comes from good health and nutrition, then not only will you look and feel so much better but people will react to you in a more positive way.

8. Finally, your skin is quite capable of making you look 20 years younger or 20 years older than your actual age, so it is worth looking after and preserving! Love yourself? Then love the skin you're in!

Chapter Two

The amazing structure of your skin and *why* it is so important to understand this

In order to get the most from this book it is vital to understand not only "**How**" but also "**Why**", and that means you being aware of the three normal layers of your skin and the functions each one has. I know that you're probably itching to get down to the nitty-gritty, but **please** remember what I said and **do not skip this section** – it is included for a very good reason and will greatly enhance your understanding of, and the likelihood of you sticking with, the plan in the long term.

It is also information that the big skincare companies would prefer you did not know, as it helps you to make an informed decision over which products you

do not want to put on your skin. You will find many references back to this information in later chapters.

So, your skin has three main functions which are:

- **Protection**
- **Regulation**
- **Sensation**

It is your body's main barrier against injury and disease, its main role being to generally reject any extraneous substances that try to pass through it. It provides **protection** therefore, from mechanical impacts and pressure, micro-organisms, radiation, chemicals and general pollution.

It is, however, a permeable membrane which, whilst blocking the majority of substances from crossing its barrier, can selectively allow others to pass through it (a process known as Trans-dermal Absorption) and which is also instrumental in eliminating a certain amount of waste and toxins from inside your body via its surface pores, through sweating. In a way this is a sort of reverse protection in that it allows the body another outlet through which to get rid of its waste products.

It **regulates** your body temperature via sweat and hair and is also responsible, through sweat, for regulating changes in your peripheral (surface) circulation and the essential balance of fluids in your body.

It empowers you with the **sensations** of touch and pressure, transmitted through an extensive network of specialized nerve cells that detect changes in the environment and relay this vital information to the brain. There are separate receptors for heat, cold, touch and pain.

All of these functions take place via specialist cells, nerves, blood vessels and glands that are present in the outer and middle layers of the skin, the **Epidermis** and the **Dermis** respectively. Both of these vary in thickness on different parts of your body, for example the epidermis, or outer layer, is thinnest on the eyelids and thickest on the palms of your hands and the soles of your feet.

The dermis is, in general, around four times thicker than the epidermis and in between the two layers is something called the **Dermal-Epidermal Junction**, a vitally important feature that interlocks to form finger-like projections called **Rete Ridges.** The purpose of these is to increase that area of the epidermis which receives essential nutrients from the blood vessels deep within the dermis.

The third – or basal – layer of your skin is simply called the **Subcutaneous Tissue**, and it is made up of connective tissue and fat which houses the larger blood vessels and nerves. The fat cells supply your body with insulation, and are also what help to give your skin a lovely full and plump appearance.

So how is the epidermis formed, and what does it do?

The function of this outer layer of your skin is to protect its inner layers from any "nasties" thrown at it by the environment! The epidermis in itself has five layers, which gives you some idea of the complexity of this, the largest organ in your body. However there is no need for you to know any but the very outer layer, the **stratum corneum** (or horny layer!).

This toughened texture of your outer skin is caused by the continual movement of **keratinocytes** (the epidermal cells) from the basal layer of the epidermis where they begin their life cycle as young living cells, to the surface where they flatten and die. This process is called **cornification.**

Once the keratinocytes reach the surface they form a hard, protective layer that is continually being worn away or "shed" (hence the nickname "horny layer"!). We women often like to give this process a helping hand through regular exfoliation, a process which stimulates cell renewal through the removal of dead skin cells and leaves the surface of our skin looking smoother, brighter and better primed to absorb our current moisturizer/facial cream of choice.

With regard to exfoliation, and as I don't want you to do anything that will remotely interfere with the success of "The Plan", I must just point out that as with many things, too much can be harmful to your skin in the long term and unfortunately, at the same time as you are sloughing away your dead skin cells you may also be removing natural oils which are vital to help protect and repair your skin. Over a period of time this could be a contributory factor to, for example dehydration, broken blood vessels and thinning skin that will eventually sag and wrinkle. So be gentle and sparing with this process, especially if you have sensitive skin and do not want to cause undue redness, sensitivity and irritation.

One thing I learnt as a nurse is that once we start interfering with the natural processes in our bodies, our bodies become lazy and less efficient in response. If you slather moisturizer onto your skin day in, day out, then your body will register this and eventually see no further need to continue producing its own natural oils.

Sometimes it really is important to accept that nature knows best and that some of the things we do to try to slow down our skin's natural ageing process can actually end up by having completely the opposite effect.

Incidentally, the keratin that is the nucleus (or core) of every epidermal cell is also the protein from which hair and nails are formed. It helps maintain your skin's resistance to physical wear and tear and also makes it waterproof (rather essential, wouldn't you say?!).

Finally, within its layers the epidermis contains three types of *specialized* cells. **Langerhans cells** are the frontline defense of your skin's immune system. **Melanocytes** produce the pigment melanin which protects from UV radiation and gives your skin its colour, and the third group, the **Merkel Cells**, is thought to be instrumental in the process of touch.

OK, so what about the dermis?

As your skin's middle layer, the dermis contains its structural elements, which are many different types of **connective tissue**. Each type of connective tissue has a different function, and this is where it gets interesting for us as three prime examples are **collagen**, **glycosaminoglycans** and **elastin**.

These three substances form the foundation of your skin, a bit like a new sofa that is firm and springy to the touch but with wear and tear becomes saggy and loses its bounce. They are of vital importance in giving your skin its strength, turgor (the state of tension or fullness in its cells due to high water content) and elasticity, and the efforts of skincare companies to replace them in ageing skin is a never-ending challenge which they have yet to overcome successfully.

As we become older, a gradual decrease in the production of these substances in our bodies is normal as part of the ageing process. However the process will be accelerated *a hundred-fold* by other factors such as poor diet, smoking, excessive alcohol consumption, dangerous levels of sun exposure, pollution and medication (in particular steroidal drugs)

27

to name but a few! All of these will contribute towards further weakening the fibres of collagen and elastin in your body, resulting in prematurely thin, fragile skin that will sag, wrinkle and become prone to bruising. Do you want me to go on? I admit I'm purposely trying to scare you here, because it's that fear that is going to kick-start you into action. Nevertheless the facts, unlike today's airbrushed celebrity photographs, do not lie.

Apart from the all-important connective tissue, the dermis also contains the following within its two layers:

a. **Hair Follicles:** these are like little sheaths in which hairs grow. The hairs play an important part in temperature regulation.

b. **Sebaceous Glands:** these glands produce oil called *sebum* which keeps the hairs clean and free from dust and bacteria.

c. **Sweat Glands:** these produce sweat which travels via sweat ducts to tiny openings in your epidermis called *pores*, and this whole ingenious little system is, again, vital to temperature regulation and elimination.

d. **Blood Vessels and Nerves:** these transmit sensations such as touch, pressure, pain, itching, heat or cold.

With me so far? Great! Now go back and read this section as many times as you need to, to fully absorb and understand the facts. This information is powerful stuff and it will be invaluable to you in your understanding of **how and why** your skin ages, and why the key to "holding back the years" is actually a very simple and logical one. You would also be surprised at how few people actually know about or indeed understand the relevance of, the information you have just been reading.

Chapter Three

What are wrinkles and what causes them?

Firstly it is necessary to realize that you cannot measure yourself by others, be it celebrities, family, friends or the impossibly gorgeous stranger you couldn't take your eyes off on the beach in Barbados while on holiday!

It is important to understand that we all have three different ages, one of which is obviously our **Chronological Age**, namely the number of years since we were born.

Then there is our **Psychological Age** which is how old we actually feel. Someone of 30 in poor health or with a lot of problems or responsibilities may feel twice their age, whereas a person in their 70s who is fit, active and healthy may *feel* only 55!

Crucially, then, is our **Biological Age** which is how well our body looks and performs at any given time and this depends on many factors such as our genes, overall health, diet and life-style, nationality or the country we live in. Again, someone of 30 who is in poor health or has grossly abused their health may look twenty years older than their chronological age, whereas someone in their 70s who has looked after themselves, has good health, a young, modern outlook and good genes (any combination of these factors) may have a biological age of around only 60.

Your skin **will,** at some point, develop wrinkles as your chronological age advances and the natural ageing process kicks in, and this is an inescapable fact of life which you have to accept. However as I mentioned in earlier chapters, your skin is a transparent mirror of diet and lifestyle so sagging and wrinkles can also be signs that your skin is not in tip-top condition. This said, there is much you can do to delay both the onset and the severity of skin ageing, and to ensure that your biological age is the best it can possibly be throughout every stage of your life.

When you see a young baby, do you ever notice its skin? It is pure, perfect, not a line or wrinkle in sight, like a blank canvas waiting to be imprinted by the masterly, artistic hand of life's experience. This completely natural process begins as soon as we leave the womb, and is something we all have to go through as the wheel of our life slowly begins to turn. I will be explaining the major contributing factors of ageing and wrinkles very shortly, *but first I want you to understand **how and why** lines and wrinkles develop in your once flawless skin*.

Wrinkles – which are basically creases on the surface of your skin – can present as either fine surface lines or deep, feature-changing furrows, dependent on the cause, the degree of development, and to a certain extent on your genetic make-up. The process is in part due to your advancing chronological age, and in part due to other contributing factors such as the lifestyle choices you make.

As your chronological age advances, the cells in your epidermis will undergo changes. Not only do they decrease at a rate of 10% per decade, but they start to divide more slowly which means your skin is not able to repair itself as efficiently. They also become thinner and less "tacky" so that moisture is less able to be retained. This causes dryness, a condition that creates a breeding ground for lines and wrinkles both on your face and on your body.

"Wherever your skin is dry, wrinkles will eventually occur"

I cannot stress this enough, **Good hydration** is absolutely crucial both to your overall health (it transports nutrients to the cells, flushes out toxins and eliminates waste), and to the health, texture and appearance of your skin. Being fully hydrated will smooth the surface of your skin in much the same way that a basic moisturizer will do. Plus it will cost much less and last much longer.

Many years ago and before I began working nights, I went to Weight Watchers in a last ditch attempt to lose some weight. This was a long time before the current Pro-Points plan (overall not as good in my opinion, as you can live on fish and chips and Danish pastries every day so long as you don't exceed your points).

Apart from the emphasis on plenty of fresh fruit and veggies the "then" diet required you to maintain a minimum intake of eight glasses of water a day. I remember groaning inwardly at the thought (I was not big on drinking water and preferred wine) but did as I was told anyway, and not only did I lose weight but my skin looked and felt the best it had in almost my entire life. It was smooth, virtually flawless, and it glowed. And if you don't believe me you only have to run a search on the internet to find pages and pages of evidence that dry skin not only causes wrinkles but more than **doubles** the speed at which they develop.

Being interested in researching such things, I have read recently about a study that ran over eight years, results of which have been published in the British Journal of Dermatology. It shows that, for a typical 28 year old woman with dry skin, the amount of visible wrinkles will have increased by a massive 52% by the time she reaches 36. However were she to keep her skin well hydrated **from the inside** with water, her wrinkles at the same age would only increase by 22%.

Even thus far, I'm sure I don't now need to say that to temporarily re-hydrate the cells on the surface of your skin with moisturizing creams is not enough and is not what this book is about. However you will now be aware of what happens naturally to the cells of your skin's surface layers as your body becomes older, and this understanding is half the battle.

Meanwhile, not to be outdone, down in the dermis as I mentioned previously, there is a natural decrease in the production of collagen. And as if that were not enough the elastin fibres start to wear out. As these natural substances are responsible for your skin's strength and elasticity this decrease is a major, contributory factor to wrinkly, saggy skin.

Also, if you remember we learned about the *rete ridges* that lie in between the dermis and the epidermis. Well, these finger-like projections will eventually start to flatten out, meaning that fewer and fewer vital nutrients are able to be transported to the epidermis from the larger blood vessels deep within the skin. I almost forgot to mention here that you will also have a reduction in the number of sweat glands which, as sweating helps to oxygenate the skin and give it a healthy glow, further contributes towards dryness and potential wrinkles.

And finally, buried deep in the subcutaneous layer, your skin's fat cells will gradually become thinner – yet another natural process that occurs as you get older and that leads to even more wrinkles/visible signs of ageing.

All these processes I have described will happen naturally in your body as a result of the passing of time, and no-one is exempt. However the transformation generally happens slowly and gradually, and nowadays there has never been a better time for people to have access to information and products that can help turn back that clock and make the absolute best of themselves for as long as they are able throughout their lifetime.

Chapter Four

Circulation and your skin – this connection is *vital*

I have chosen to give this topic a section all to itself as good circulation is the fundamental key to all your health and beauty issues, and is the basic concept around which this book has evolved.

I think most people are aware these days, of the dangers of clogging up their arteries, something that can impact on their health in the most devastating way by massively increasing the risk of heart attacks or a stroke. Many people however, do not realize the effect of bad circulation upon their skin, both directly, and also indirectly as a result of other circulatory-related health issues.

Consider these two statements:

a. A leading cause of ageing is the body's increasing inability to get oxygen into its cells.

b. The skin is a living organ which needs to be constantly supplied with oxygen and nutrients carried from the bloodstream and without which it will shrivel and die.

Circulation refers quite simply to the flow of blood around your body to and from the heart (which is like a muscular pump divided into four chambers), and this continuous circuit is called the **Systemic Circulation.** Without giving you another detailed biology lesson, this process happens in two steps as follows:

Step 1: oxygen-depleted blood is transported to the right sided chambers of the heart by the two largest veins in the body, the venae cavae. From here it is pumped into the pulmonary artery and carried to the lungs where it loses its carbon dioxide and picks up fresh oxygen.

Step 2: this oxygen and nutrient-rich blood then returns to the left side of the heart where it is pumped into the largest artery in the body, the aorta. It is then transported, via a complex and microscopic arterial system, throughout the rest of your body to your tissues, muscles and all your vital organs including your skin, picking up carbon dioxide and waste products for excretion on its way so that the whole cycle then begins all over again.

The 5 litres of blood contained in the blood vessels of a typical adult complete this circuit in just under a minute. Think about this for a moment. Your blood circulates around your body 1500 times every single day without stopping (in normal circumstances), for the duration of your lifetime - an absolutely amazing feat of engineering.

Earlier I talked about how a baby's skin is so perfectly flawless when it is born, and before being exposed to pollution and all the other "nasties" that life throws at it. You are also blessed at birth with a squeaky clean circulatory system – your blood vessels are wide and clear and your blood flows easily around your body with no resistance. This is rather like a brand new car that is such a joy to drive because the engine and all system components are shiny and new, and oil and fuel flow freely through an unclogged system.

Even into early adult-hood your body remains young and strong, replete with a plentiful and uninterrupted flow of oxygen and vital nutrients to its cells. Then, slowly and insidiously the rot starts to set in as the natural ageing process combined with all the undesirable habits we acquire (be they active or passive) sees the start of a build-up of toxins and fatty deposits in our once perfect system. Our blood vessels start to acquire deposits of plaque on the inside and become narrowed and, as a result, our heart has to work harder to pump the same amount of blood through the increasingly gunged-up pipes of our circulatory system.

So what does this mean for our skin?

Well, as our circulation is the holistic link between every system and organ in our body, it means that as it becomes more sluggish, our muscles, tissues and vital organs – including our skin– are little by little being deprived of the life-giving oxygen, glucose and nutrients that they need to operate efficiently.

Inflammation sets in which further inhibits the flow of blood around the body. I am not talking here about the more positive type of inflammation that is your body's natural and temporary response to injury (for example, a sprain, a rash, a sore throat etc) but the hidden, chronic inflammation that attacks your immune system and impairs its ability to function – a reaction triggered by exposure since birth to pollution, chemicals and synthetic and processed foods.

This more sinister form is, I firmly believe, the cause of all the chronic illnesses and diseases that may afflict us in our lifetime, with links to coronary heart disease, cardiovascular disease, cancer, diabetes, neurological disorders and auto-immune disorders. It results in damage and/or destruction of body cells and tissues, and has a devastating effect not only on our entire system but specifically on our skin through its response to chronic illness and disease, and the ensuing build-up of free radicals which causes rapid ageing. We cannot see inside our bodies, we do not see this process start to happen. Our first inkling is when we begin to notice changes in the way our body functions, or in our looks.

I used to work on a Rheumatology Unit nursing patients who were severely crippled with arthritis and struggling to move around on their painful, inflamed joints - the point being that their disability (with strong links as we have seen, to poor circulation and the ensuing inflammation and pain that this generates) inhibits their ability to move around. This in turn slows down the circulation even further, which has a devastating effect on internal organs and, very visibly, the skin. A vicious circle of events to ponder …

Now while I'm not suggesting that you will necessarily be afflicted by any of the conditions mentioned above - after all many people are lucky enough to go through life and remain relatively healthy – I hope you can now see that Good Health = Good Skin, and that if you want to keep your good health and hold onto your lovely skin for as long as possible (or on the other hand if you have problem skin and want to improve it), then *you need to take immediate action to keep your circulation flowing freely through a healthy system that is not clogged up with gunge*. I cannot stress enough how important this is. So please, if you remember nothing else remember this:-

"a sluggish and inefficient circulation is the root of all your health and beauty issues."

The causes of poor circulation are many, but can mostly be traced back to lifestyle choices such as poor diet, namely refined flours, sugar, trans-fats and processed foods, lack of exercise, smoking, drinking, stress – in fact all of the "deadly sins" that I'm about to tell you will wreak havoc on your skin. This is logical if you think about it, as bad skin is a by-product of bad circulation.

Yes we are constantly being told that to smoke is bad for our skin, which is absolutely true, but the basic underlying reason **why** it is so bad is that it gradually narrows your blood vessels by causing a build up of plaque which impedes the flow of blood around your body, and it is this, this increasingly inefficient circulation, that kills your skin by gradually starving it of the oxygen and nutrients that it needs to survive.

Read this again and again if you need to, because for this plan to work for you, the knowledge and understanding of **How** and **Why** is as important as the actual plan itself.

In Summary

1. We all have three different ages- **Chronological**, **Psychological** and **Biological**. Your biological age is how well your body looks and performs at any given stage of your life regardless of your chronological age, and this is the one we are most concerned with. Your psychological age is how old you actually feel.

2. You are born with a perfect, flawless skin and a circulatory system that works like a well-oiled machine. *So what happens?*

3. As your Chronological age advances, the natural process of ageing inevitably kicks in – your epidermal cells decrease at a rate of 10%

39

per decade, their rate of renewal is less efficient and they become thinner and less "tacky", resulting in moisture loss and dry skin. There is a marked decrease of collagen and elastin in the dermis, which means that your skin loses some of its strength and elasticity. In addition your *rete ridges* start to flatten out, your *sweat glands* start to decrease in number, and the *fat cells* in the subcutaneous layer of your skin become thinner. The effect of all this may be seen quite early on in some people, while others may not notice any significant changes until well into middle age.

4. The rate at which this natural ageing process occurs **will accelerate a hundred fold** in response to other factors, largely the lifestyle choices that you make, for example poor diet, smoking, excessive alcohol consumption and excessive sun exposure (full list to follow shortly!).

5. Remember that dry skin more than doubles the rate at which wrinkles may develop, so **it is vital to hydrate your skin from the inside** with at least eight glasses of water a day. Whatever you may read to the contrary, your body depends on it. And Finally …

PoorDiet/Smoking/Alcohol/SunExposure/Stress/Toxins/ Chemicals and Lack of Exercise

equal

Inefficient Circulation

which leads to

Chronic Inflammation

which results in

Increasing Health Problems and an Ageing, Unhealthy Skin

I hope that you can now see without a shadow of a doubt, that the secret to youthful, radiant skin on the outside simply **must** come from within. It is, as they say, a "no-brainer".

Chapter Five

Anti-Oxidants and Free Radicals clearly explained

Many of you will have heard of anti-oxidants and free radicals, however as they are yet another vital link in the chain of all things important to the internal health approach, I'm including a brief overview to clarify the importance of their role in your body's ageing process.

Every one of the trillions of cells in your body is made up of **Molecules** and each molecule contains one or more **Atoms** bonded together by **Electrons**.

Electrons are negatively charged particles that occur *in pairs* for normal cell activity and normally these paired bonds don't split. However when weak bonds *do* split the molecule, sadly, is left with an odd number of electrons and becomes a **Free Radical** (a bit like losing a partner or best friend!).

A **Free Radical** (so called because it wanders or "floats" around in its search for stability) is a molecule with an unpaired electron, desperately looking to stabilize itself by "stealing" an electron from a normal molecule. In its search for that extra electron, a free radical can become highly rebellious and unstable. It will attack the nearest stable molecule which will then itself have an unpaired electron and become a free radical, so setting in motion a chain reaction that, if unchecked, will cause irreparable damage and destruction. In your body this snowball effect can wreak devastation on the healthy living cells of, for example, heart muscle, nerves, your immune system and your skin.

Free Radicals are a by-product of detoxifying processes, and they are everywhere both in your body and in the world around you. They cause deterioration through oxidation, not only of body cells and tissues but of everyday materials such as paint, plastics, works of art, foodstuffs etc. Whether fading paint or sliced apple turned brown, this deterioration is entirely due to free radical activity.

Most free radicals exist only for a nano-second, but it is the chain reaction that each sets in motion that is so damaging as it will continue to spiral out of control until an anti-oxidant scavenges the offending free radical without itself becoming reactive or unstable. This breaks the chain, thus terminating the reaction before more vital molecules are damaged.

I just used an example of an apple turning brown: an effective antidote to this is to sprinkle lemon juice over the flesh of the apple once sliced, to ensure that it stays white. This happens because lemon juice is an anti-oxidant - it generously "donates" its electron to prevent damage from the free radicals produced by the apple upon exposure to the atmosphere. Amazing to think of all this activity going on in the world around us, isn't it!

In your body there are small numbers of free radicals present all the time and your body's defense system normally acts to keep the numbers small. In fact those produced from the immune system are considered beneficial as they destroy bacteria and viruses. We also need a certain amount of free radicals to produce substances such as hormones and enzymes (essential to the proper functioning of our bodies), to generate energy, and to help increase the blood flow in response to a stressful situation.

However over a period of time, and in response to factors such as age, poor diet, smoking and pollution, your body will produce more free radicals than it does scavengers (in the form of anti-oxidants) to control them. And when this state of emergency is reached then the pathways to ageing and disease will be wide open.   The resulting cell damage presents on the outside with wrinkles, sagging and dull, unresponsive skin (like the browning flesh of the apple on exposure to air) and internally by creating a state of inflammation (our old friend!) with all its associated and devastating problems.

Free radicals can even damage the particles in your blood, further contributing to a build up of plaque in your blood vessels (and we have seen what irreparable damage that can cause). As I mentioned before, everything in your body is to do with **Balance** … you need both free radicals and anti-oxidants, but if the natural balance isn't right then your body will suffer nasty structural changes as a result. This is why it is far better to work on removing as many toxins as you can from your life, and to take your anti-oxidants from a natural dietary source rather than from overdosing on vast amounts of anti-oxidant vitamins which can actually block your body's natural ability to control itself.

So What Else Disrupts This Balance?

Well there are several reasons why your body will produce an excess of Free Radicals. They increase naturally in your body with *age*, and as a direct result of exposure from birth, to *pollutants, toxins* and *chemicals*, and *junk food*. They will multiply at an alarming rate in response to *tobacco smoke, alcohol, sugary and processed foods, car fumes* and *radiation* (both from sun exposure and from x rays). A *high fat diet* (in particular fried foods) will also accelerate the process, as ***fat molecules can create oxidation***.

Other factors contributing to the creation of free radicals are *stress* and, bizarrely enough, *strenuous exercise,* although exercise can also actually increase your body's anti-oxidant activities to compensate, so once again it is all about ***Balance!***

Always remember that you are the "face" of what you eat and that your diet can be your best friend or your worst enemy!

And How Exactly Do Anti-Oxidants Help?

Anti-Oxidants are molecules found in vitamins, minerals and other nutrients sourced from the food we eat, and/or supplements. They are your body's natural defense system – the "good guys" that will safely interact with a free radical to interrupt the chain reaction I talked about earlier, **before** vital molecules are damaged. They have the ability to give up one of their electrons without themselves undergoing any change, so are completely self-sacrificing! And you will find many of them in the most colourful **fruits and vegetables** – red, yellow and orange, purple, green and blue.

The principle anti-oxidants are **vitamin C**, **vitamin E, beta carotene** (a precursor to vitamin A or retinol), **selenium** and **zinc**. The body cannot manufacture these so you need to replenish them in your body every day through diet and/or supplements.

You should be able to get all the nutrients you need from a balanced and varied diet (moreover, anti-oxidants from this source are better absorbed by the body), but if you are at high risk of free radical damage or you have a known vitamin or mineral deficiency, then you may need supplements in addition (in which case remember that powders and liquids absorb much better than pills). Do be aware that *an excess of any one vitamin can deplete the levels of another* so ask advice if you are unsure.

I will be talking a lot more about anti-oxidants in Part 2, but here are some examples (not exhaustive by any means) of the types of food in which they are to be found, and the RDA (Recommended Daily Amount for an average healthy person) as per the UK's NHS guidelines. The RDA from large manufacturers is usually around double this amount (my rather cynical opinion is that this is because they want you to buy twice as much!) so if you really feel the need to use supplements then maybe somewhere in between would be a good point to aim for.

Vitamin C (ascorbic acid) is a water soluble vitamin that is found in berries, citrus fruit and juices, grapefruit, kiwi, cantaloupe, green peppers, sprouts, cauliflower, spinach, broccoli and sweet potatoes. It is unable to be stored in the body so needs to be replenished daily. *RDA = 40mg.*

Vitamin E (d-alpha tocopherol) is a fat soluble vitamin found in nuts, seeds, vegetable and fish oils, whole grains (especially wheatgerm), fortified cereals, berries, apricots, pumpkin, red peppers, broccoli, carrots and spinach. This vitamin needs a certain amount of fat in the diet to help in its absorption, and any excess is able to be stored by the body. *RDA = 3mg for men, 4mg for women.*

Beta Carotene is present in carrots, squash, broccoli, yams, spinach, beets, asparagus, sweet potato, mango, apricots, pink grapefruit, peaches, cantaloupe, tomatoes and grains. Tomatoes in particular, are extremely high in an anti-oxidant called *lycopene* which, incidentally, gives them their customary red colour …

Not only does lycopene fight against free radicals and protect your skin from UV rays but it also helps prevent the break-down of collagen in your skin, guarding against loss of elasticity and the ensuing development of wrinkles. Because beta carotene is converted into vitamin A by the body there is no set daily requirement, although if taken in excess as a supplement, vitamin A in itself can be quite toxic. Also it has no anti-oxidant properties.

Selenium is a trace metal present in brazil nuts, tuna, beef, poultry, eggs and fortified breads. *RDA = 0.075mg for men, 0.06 mg for women.*

Zinc is mostly found in meat, shellfish, milk and other dairy produce such as cheese, bread and cereal products and wheatgerm. *RDA = 5.5-9.5mg for men, 4-7mg for women …*

… which brings this chapter (rather longer than I intended!) to an end. I hope you now understand more fully **why** so much importance is attached to the devastating effect that an imbalance of free radicals can have on your skin and the ageing process in general: how and why they cause plaque build-up and contribute massively to poor circulation and chronic inflammation: and how **the power to break this chain of destruction lies in your hands and your hands alone**. You do this by:

a. Eliminating from your life all the factors that actively produce free radicals.
b. Providing your body with the means to fight them through a diet rich in delicious foods just bursting with anti-oxidants to repair and protect your skin. It is *that* simple. I promise you will be delighted by the results!

This brings us neatly to the final chapter in this section, a summing up of the deadliest enemies of your skin, each and every one of which is a major contributor to the ageing process and will result in a sluggish and inefficient circulation, chronic inflammation, excessive free radical formation and, ultimately, dehydrated, wrinkly and saggy skin. Indulge at your peril!

Chapter Six

15 Deadly Enemies of your Skin: *why* and *how* they have such a massive impact upon ageing

Smoking is possibly the worst form of suicide for your skin, and a major accelerator of the natural ageing process. It is also fast acting, as a young person who starts smoking between 15 and 20 can be showing the first signs of skin damage *before the age of 30.*

Smoking kills your skin by slowly starving the outermost layer (or epidermis) of vital oxygen and nutrients, among them vitamin C, vitamin E and the immunity-boosting vitamin A. It does this by very gradually narrowing the blood vessels throughout your body, so that oxygen and nutrients can no longer be transported efficiently to the cells. Over a period of time this leads to the formation and build-up of harmful free radicals, which in turn damages the elastin fibres that keep your skin strong and supple. Inevitably this results in the appearance of fine lines and premature wrinkles.

The efficient transport of oxygen around your body is further impeded by a depletion of folic acid, which, along with vitamin B12, works to facilitate this process. In addition, your body's natural defenses are slowly weakened as they are constantly being called upon to deal with the harmful chemicals contained in the smoke you inhale from each cigarette.

Smoking also stains your teeth and nails, turning them yellow (a most unattractive look) and over time will weaken and rot them.

The message therefore, is loud and clear … if you want to recover or maintain your vital, youthful appearance and enjoy an amazing and healthy old age, you need to think seriously about giving smoking up for good - as every cigarette you have will cancel out the beneficial effects of an otherwise healthy diet and lifestyle and can (according to recent research) shorten your life by an average 10 -11 minutes. **Even just one cigarette a day** has the potential to treble your risk of heart disease.

Alcohol is another major offender. It has a similar effect to that of smoking in that it depletes the body of vitamin A (the only skincare ingredient that the US Food and Drug Administration recognizes as truly anti-ageing). This means that your skin's natural defense system is lowered, making it easier for toxic, harmful substances to pass through the skin into your body.

Vitamin A is also used in your skin's turnover process – the outer layer of skin is continually sloughing off dead cells as new ones take their place, but if your skin is suffering then this process happens less and less frequently. As a result your skin begins to look dull and lack lustre – and it is at this point that many women start thinking of using an exfoliation product which, as I mentioned earlier, will only serve to exacerbate this problem in the long term.

Alcohol also dilates the blood vessels every time you have a drink, and eventually they will remain permanently dilated and lose their tone. This of course has a drastic impact upon your circulation which becomes sluggish and inefficient, and you should by now be acutely aware of the seriously damaging and far-reaching consequences that this will have.

Excessive drinking can also lead to chronic dilation of the smaller capillaries on the surface of your skin and a permanent flush on your face, and for these reasons you can see how alcohol also worsens conditions such as acne and rosacea (a skin disorder which presents with redness, flushing, pimples and pus-heads). As with smoking, and indeed as with most of the "deadly sins" listed in this chapter, it can also result in a significant build-up of free radicals.

Finally, alcohol is a diuretic. Every drink you have can stimulate your body to pass around four times as much urine, which will result in dehydration and associated dry and lifeless-looking skin.

Bad Fats Even though we are constantly told to avoid fats in our everyday diet, it is important to realize that some fats are essential for our general well-being and for the health and radiance of our skin, *ie* it is the type of fat and the amount we eat of it that matters.

As well as being an important source of energy, fat is vital in maintaining your mental function and preventing fatigue. It is a source of certain vitamins such as vitamin A and vitamin D, also essential fatty acids that your body is unable to make for itself … plus it helps your body absorb certain nutrients which is why low fat diets are a killer for your overall health and for your skin. It is so easy for big weight-loss companies to market to the majority of people who don't understand what these diets are doing to their bodies.

For years we have been led to believe that it is **saturated fats** which are the real "baddies" (those found in animal products such as meat, whole milk, butter and cheese) - and yes it is true that these fats, in excess, can raise your cholesterol levels and contribute to the build-up of plaque in your arteries, resulting in poor circulation - part of the chain of events we have been talking about that causes ageing skin and the risk of heart disease.

They may also contribute to the worsening of any inflammatory skin condition such as acne, eczema and psoriasis.

They should therefore be eaten in very moderate amounts, a maximum of **20g/day** for women and **30g/day** for men and as part of a balanced diet rich in antioxidants from fresh fruit and vegetables. *Do not* make the mistake of cutting them out of your diet completely, however, as your body needs a certain amount of these fats for several reasons. These include having an anti-viral effect on harmful bacteria and viruses, helping in the absorption of several important vitamins and minerals such as vitamins A, D, E, K and calcium, and preserving the tension in cell membranes, thus increasing immunity against virus attacks.

As I have said before it is all about **Balance** and **Harmony** within the body … eliminate one essential group of foodstuffs from your diet and this balance will be disturbed, with consequences.

Unfortunately, due to the understandably bad press that saturated fats have received – namely that they cause dangerously high levels of cholesterol with all its associated health risks - many people have tried to avoid them altogether by taking low fat substitutes that are not real or whole foods and that have few, if any, redeeming health benefits.

Our bodies actually *need* a certain amount of *cholesterol* to assist with the manufacture of hormones and as an important part of the composition of our skin, and as only a very small proportion of the cholesterol in our blood comes from food then it would seem that saturated fats are not quite the ogres that they are made out to be, and certainly not when compared to the dangers of eating foods with a high sugar content.

Trans Fats on the other hand, pose a far more sinister risk, and are very ugly indeed. They are formed when a vegetable oil is changed from a liquid (as found naturally) to a solid … a process known as **Hydrogenation.** This term is used to describe any process where a product has been biochemically altered using hydrogenated fats, for instance in the manufacture of "low-fat" or "easy-spread" alternatives to butter. *Trans Fatty Acids are the by-products of this ruinous process…altered compounds which are seriously detrimental to your health in that, as well as being linked irrevocably to high cholesterol and heart disease (they are unable to be broken down in the body) they cause oxidation (one of the major causes of free radical formation) and will in fact actively promote inflammation and worsen any existing skin condition.*

The Government in this country has unfortunately not yet supported a full ban on trans fats in food products, and so long as vendors selling *unpackaged* foods are not obliged by law to list their ingredients it is almost impossible to know the amount of trans fats that are present. The worst culprits have long been fast food chains which are currently being allowed to decrease the amount of hydrogenated (or partially hydrogenated) oils in their products as they see fit. Producers of *packaged* foods did agree to stop using these as ingredients, but in fact several foods still include them (look for "*mono* and d*iglycerides of fatty acids*" in the "what is contained" list.

Basically trans fats are to be found in processed foods, almost every take-away meal you eat, fried foods, bought cakes and pastries, biscuits, bread and ice cream.

Ideally you should eat no more than around **5g/day** of trans-fats but as I already mentioned it is very difficult to even estimate the amount you are consuming, so all you can do is just attempt to eat as few of these foods as possible.

Always read carefully, the labels on all packaged and processed foods in order to avoid them. Learn how to make informed and healthy choices that will have long-term benefits for your health and well-being. Focus upon the good fats, moderate the saturated fats, and eliminate as many trans fats from your diet as you can. Your skin will love you for it!

GoodFats fall into three categories: *monounsaturated fats*, *polyunsaturated fats* and *omega 3s* which, as we have seen, play a vital role in fighting fatigue and in improving mental function. In contrast to saturated fats and trans-fats they will actually lower your cholesterol and decrease your risk of heart disease, plus they are good for your overall health, and your skin loves them! They can be found in foods such as avocados, nuts and seeds, fatty fish like salmon, sardines, tuna, mackerel or herring, tofu, olives, olive oil and sunflower oil.

Of course you need to control your intake even of these good fats, as you may put on weight if, for example, you eat vast quantities of nuts on a regular basis. So again, aim for around **10-15%** of your daily calorific intake. Once, however, you have read the following section on the dastardly effects that sugar has on your body, you will realize that the real enemy in today's modern world, the one that is up there at the top of the list of things that are a killer for your health and your skin, is not fat but is indeed sugar. Read on ...

Sugar
It is now recognized that an excess of sugar in our diet has far greater detrimental effects on our general health and well-being as does to consume too much saturated fat. Its dangers are up there on a par with smoking and excessive alcohol consumption. As a nation we are addicted to it as a quick fix to boost energy levels and generally make us feel better. It "helps" us cope with the stress and strain of everyday life, and is also addictive in that one square of chocolate will leave us wanting – and needing – more.

This is because sugar has a similar effect to other addictive substances such as heroin, in that it releases "feel good" chemicals in the brain that cause us to want to repeat the experience.

Supermarkets are well aware of this fact, and cash in on it quite unashamedly by placing stands of chocolate and other sugary snacks at their checkouts (a ploy that has been shown to boost sales by over 50%). They exploit the fact that, having already filled their trolley with all sorts of goodies and treats that they probably didn't even come in for, by the time they reach checkout customers are in maximum buying mode and most likely to think "Mmm, I've spent all this money, might as well grab a bar of chocolate"!

It's all about **mind games,** a sneaky trick by our canny supermarkets to boost their profits - and most of us have fallen for it at one time or another! Petrol Stations too: I was waiting in a queue to pay for my petrol only this morning, flanked entirely down one side by chocolate bars three stands deep. Of the five people in front of me, two took a bar of chocolate as they passed, and one a packet of crisps - and everyone was being asked at the till if they wanted to "take advantage of our special offers on chocolate or fizzy drinks". Of course, the argument would be that everybody has the choice to say "No", but if the merest whiff of a chocolate bar is enough to make your willpower turn to jelly then this blatant display of temptation could be seen as really irresponsible by the companies that encourage it.

A further temptation is **restaurant menus,** in particular the dessert section! Descriptions such as "sumptuous lemon pudding topped with whipped cream and crushed meringue, drizzled with a tangy lemon sauce and served with dairy vanilla ice cream" or "rich and indulgent, golden ginger sponge pudding, oozing with a delicious rum/ginger sauce and served hot with custard" (may have gone a bit overboard here!) are almost impossible to resist! But of course, as totally delicious as they sound, most of these irresistible puddings are loaded with processed sugar and fat and as such have almost zero nutritional benefit for your skin.

Packaged meals too, are guilty of using cleverly worded descriptions in order to make them sound irresistible and persuade you to buy – a similar type of advertising to that used by big skincare companies for face-creams and the like. You really do have to ignore this and read the labels to discover the sugar and fat content of everything you purchase.

The thing is with sugar, **it is almost always found in combination with "bad fats"**. You rarely get one without the other, and it is this unholy alliance between the two that reportedly has a similar effect on your brain to heroin or cocaine and that makes certain foods so addictive.

Think about it, it is a marriage made in hell! Take either food-group out of the equation and suddenly your lovely pudding, your ice-cream or your eagerly anticipated bar of chocolate doesn't taste so lovely any more. The processed food industry is well aware of this fact, and exploits it for all it is worth, even now sneakily adding extra sugar to *low fat* foods so they will taste as good and people will buy them (beware too, of *low fat/low sugar* products which will almost certainly contain artificial sweeteners such as aspartame). It is an uncompromising industry, and one where you really and truly have nowhere to run.

The blame for this sugary addiction doesn't lie entirely at our doorstep, as for many years the message has been clear … we should be eating a low fat and high carbohydrate diet based on plenty of bread, potatoes, rice and pasta, together with our recommended "five a day" portions of fresh vegetables and fruit. What we now know is that the starch contained in these foods, also the natural substance fructose to be found in fruit, converts to sugar in our blood-stream.

And what happens to all that excess sugar that our body doesn't need? *It is turned into fat.*

And it doesn't stop there. Our supermarket shelves are piled high with "healthy" low fat products, all full of extra sugar to make them taste good in the absence of fat but which is turned into fat anyway, so where exactly is the point? A low fat muffin, for example, can contain 8-9 teaspoons of sugar – significantly more than that contained in a regular muffin - and the same pattern can be seen in low fat biscuits, yoghurts, salad dressings, soups, peanut butter and the like.

A further problem is that starchy and highly processed foods have the effect of giving us a quick "sugar fix" which sends our blood sugar levels soaring, only to plummet again a couple of hours later leaving us feeling tired, moody, irritable and in need of more sugar. This tense little scenario is responsible for stimulating the release of **Insulin**, *a known principal ageing hormone.* Insulin is your body's inbuilt defense against a sudden surge of blood sugar, and it is also instrumental in turning excess sugar in your body into fat.

Even one 360ml can of fizzy drink (containing around eight teaspoonfuls of sugar) a day can lead to stored fat around your middle, a high blood pressure and raised levels of cholesterol, all of which will increase – in fact, even double - the likelihood of life-threatening conditions such as type 2 diabetes, cancer, heart disease or a stroke - and all of which will ultimately have a devastating effect on your skin.

Here too it is all about **Balance …** there are vitamins and nutrients in fruit, for example, that are essential to the health of your skin, and also in some "starchy" foods, in particular whole meal bread and potatoes (processed, low-fat foods of course, should be avoided wherever possible, as whatever the packaging says they are no good for you).

Most vegetables and salad items too, contain between ¼ - 2tsps of *natural* sugar per serving (a large swede can contain up to 8tsps!) *yet they are such a major source of vitamins, minerals and anti-oxidants that to cut them out of your diet would be tantamount to suicide!*

However we are talking here of *excess*, and the potential pitfalls of cutting one food group from your diet then compensating by increasing your intake of another. Excess or complete deprivation of any essential food group, unless for medical reasons of course, will upset the natural mechanism of your body and trigger a chain reaction … usually one which will have unpleasant and undesired effects!

So what does sugar actually DO, that is so bad?

Well as we have seen, sugar will convert directly to fat in your body, and while it may appear to give you an energy boost this is short lived and only serves to fuel your cravings for more and more sugar. Over a period of time this will greatly increase the risk of *diabetes* and *obesity*. But it does not stop there. Not only does sugar interfere with the delicate balance of minerals in your body but it upsets the efficiency of your immune system, causes problems with your digestive tract, can result in anxiety, memory loss and a lack of concentration, can severely compromise fertility and, to top it all, has been found to have strong links to the development of Alzheimer's disease and several common forms of cancer.

And how does all this affect our skin?

The bottom line is this, that if your diet is full of sugar and starch, then your skin will suffer premature ageing and lack radiance. **Sugar is a major contributor to the AGE-producing process in your body** (of which more shortly) … sugar molecules attach to the collagen fibres in the dermal layer of your skin and react with them (a process known as *glycation*) causing a loss of turgor and elasticity which leads to sagging, wrinkles and a higher risk of sun damage. In addition, most of the health problems mentioned above will, in support of the general theme of this book, sooner or later affect the condition and luminosity of your skin. Enough said!

Excessive intake of Salt

Sea Salt is a crystalline mineral which is produced mainly from the evaporation of sea water from the world's oceans. Its main component is a single chemical compound, sodium chloride, which while essential to life can also be very harmful if taken in excess.

For thousands of years salt has been recognized as an important method of food preservation, and it is also one of our basic human tastes. It is as fundamentally important to life as are water and oxygen, and as you will see it works along with water in your body to maintain the correct level of fluid balance that is vital to every bodily function. It also helps in the smooth functioning of your nervous and immune systems and in the regulation of your body's PH factor (the delicate acid/alkaline balance that is the body's inner chemistry).

However like many things, if your taste for salt is over-indulged it can upset the chemical balance in your body and cause lasting damage. It can also have a very detrimental effect on your skin at a fundamental level.

As mentioned above, one of the main functions of salt is to regulate the water content in your body, thus playing a vital role in the state of fluid balance. Sodium molecules bind to water molecules with the result that your body will respond to an excess of salt by retaining fluid - *a prime cause of the dreaded cellulite!*

It is this attempt by your body to cope with sodium overload that causes a condition known as fluid retention, and, in more serious cases, the pooling of fluid with swelling (most commonly associated with calves, ankles and feet), called *oedema*. Both conditions will almost certainly result in a significant rise in blood pressure, and will contribute long-term to impaired circulation, clogged arteries and a dull, lifeless-looking skin that is being starved of vital nutrients and further dehydrated by the medication used to treat the conditions.

An excess of salt can also result in dizziness, muscle cramps or electrolyte imbalance, which in turn may lead to increased stress levels and disturbed sleep. Both of these factors have a very negative impact on your skin and overall health. You may not notice any adverse effects from eating too much salt in the short term, but you can be sure that, at some point in your life, one way or another, those effects will make themselves known.

A large part of your daily intake of salt – around three quarters - comes from processed and packaged foods (not least due to the sodium content of many commonly used food preservatives) rather than the amount you use in cooking or sprinkle on your meal, and unless you read the labels and act on that information, it is very easy to exceed the recommended daily amount. The NHS recommends a maximum of **6gms of salt, equating to 2.5gms of sodium**, a day, and although this can be taken as a good general guide the fact is that every individual has different needs, and these needs can vary from day to day dependent on a variety of lifestyle factors such as engaging in regular strenuous activity with the associated loss of salt from the body through sweating.

Incidentally, **sodium (Na)** is just one part of the complex, consisting of natural salt or sodium chloride (NaCl) and vitally essential trace minerals - and it is measured in a slightly different way which you need to be aware of when reading food labels.

It is also interesting to note that *reduced-fat foods generally contain more salt/sodium than their full-fat counterparts, which again improves the taste in the absence of fat. Similarly, foods with low salt/sodium content usually contain extra sugar* (added, bizarrely, to counteract the salt!), meaning of course that if they don't get you one way, they get you another! It is all about the taste, as obviously nobody is going to buy meals that are unappetizing to the palate … and Heaven Forbid that the food industry should then lose out on its profits.

However the key here is not just the amount but the **type** of salt you use. Unfortunately the kind of salt contained in processed foods and standard table salts is a refined sodium that is not only stripped of most of its essential minerals which your body needs to function, and which help to keep your blood in an alkaline state, but is loaded with chemicals and preservatives such as Aluminium. *Sodium luminosilicate* and *calcium aluminosilicate* are permitted by both the European Union (EU) and the Food and Drug Administration (FDA) of the United States, despite the fact that traces of this chemical have been linked to the development of Alzheimer's in the States.

This "refining" of the natural product is why many people are actually deficient in minerals such as potassium and magnesium which are vital to preserve the chemical balance in the body, and why it is a major contributory cause to water retention, dehydration and often a raging thirst.

So why do manufacturers go to so much trouble to rid "raw" salt of all its beneficial elements? Well as usual it all comes down to money and profits. By the time they have taken the basic commodity and stripped it, bleached it and pumped it full of preservatives and anti-caking agents, it is in a much more visually appealing state to present to the consumer, it is easier to pour or sprinkle, and it will last for ever in a kitchen cupboard. The customers are happy (if blissfully unaware), and manufacturers are assured of their profits. Happy days!

In contrast, natural unrefined sea salt, apart from the fact that it has a far meatier and more satisfying taste, actually rehydrates, and restores the natural fluid balance within your body.

Wheat and AGEs Wheat-based products can accelerate the ageing process in your body due to the fact that they have the potential to massively increase

its blood sugar levels. This action intensifies the production of Advanced Glycation End products [AGEs], one of the three most significant causes of ageing that go on inside your body, the other two as already discussed, being *Inflammation* and *Oxidation*. It does this by causing molecules of glucose to attach rather stickily to the collagen fibres in your skin (rather like a poison ivy that wraps itself around a tree and saps all the life from it), thus destroying the skin's elasticity and further contributing to the development of lines and wrinkles.

AGEs are basically useless waste substances that will accumulate particularly rapidly in response to a high blood sugar, but also to other factors such as eating excessive amounts of dairy products, red meat, and all processed, smoked or pasteurized foods, and to certain cooking methods that use a very high heat like frying, barbecuing, baking and yes, even grilling. They will clog up the blood vessels in your system to cause a major impediment to your circulation that will drastically reduce the amount of oxygen and nutrients able to be transported to your major organs, including your skin. This can result in conditions such as atherosclerosis, dementia, heart failure, kidney failure and strokes.

Wheat-based products are worse than most other foods in increasing blood sugar levels to intensify the production of AGEs, largely due to a unique variety of complex carbohydrate they contain, called *amylopectin A*. It is also reported that the browned parts of baked wheat products such as bread, toast, cereals and cakes, contain carcinogenic chemicals called *acrylamides* which, in addition to increasing the risk of developing cancer, can also significantly accelerate the ageing process.

It is due to these confirmed risk factors that I have included wheat products in this section, and also because if you haven't already done so, you will no doubt read all about it at some point either in magazine articles or on the internet. **However**, there is so much naturally occurring nutritional value to be found in unrefined and organically produced wheat products that it would seem a travesty to deprive your body of these benefits entirely.

Yeast, for example, is a known source of substances called *beta-glucans* whose properties can not only assist in the *balancing* of your blood sugar but will strengthen the inbuilt front-line defense system of your body ... whilst an average slice of whole-grain bread is rich in protein and the complex carbohydrates that are your body's most stable and reliable fuel source.

I would therefore advise that, while *an avoidance of products made from any refined and highly processed flour is strongly recommended,* a small daily portion of those foods containing natural, unrefined and whole-wheat flour will provide you with enough health benefits to justify their inclusion in your diet. It is really your choice to make. For more on this, and for some valid alternatives to wheat flour, read the relevant sections in the final part of this book.

Toxins, Chemicals and Synthetic oils

From the moment we are born, our bodies are bombarded with toxins. We cannot avoid them as they are all around us - chemicals, pesticides, aerosol sprays, plastics, processed and packaged foods, the linings of canned goods, make-up, medications, cigarette smoke, alcohol, the list just goes on and on. It is quite an interesting, if shocking, exercise to list all the toxins you expose your skin to in the bathroom first thing in the morning every day of your life! You have only to read the labels on pretty much everything you use to realize that the term "Toxic Beauty" is no figment of the imagination.

Extreme up to a point – well, perhaps … after all this is the 21st century and for the majority of people, if they were to avoid every product containing toxins they wouldn't use anything at all. However it does hopefully serve a purpose in making you aware of the more undesirable elements in the multitude of bottles, jars and sprays on your bath-room shelf.

Even an innocuous looking bar of soap will more often than not contain a substance called **sodium laurel sulphate,** aka **sodium laureth sulphate,** a known irritant derived from harsh industrial cleansers such as engine degreasers, but also routinely found in almost every soap, shampoo and toothpaste on the market. Traces of it can enter into and linger in your eyes, also - if absorbed into your system through broken skin or inadvertently swallowed in a drop of soapy water – internal organs such as your heart, lungs, liver or brain. Once inside these organs, laurel sulphate has been proven to accumulate and maintain residual levels. Also, as it is such a known irritant to the skin, any product containing it is, needless to say, an absolute no-no for anyone suffering from acne, eczema, psoriasis or other inflammatory skin complaints.

Check out also, the labels on any of the products in your household cleaning cupboard, particularly those in aerosol spray cans, to see just how many chemical or synthetic ingredients they contain.

The most lethal are probably drain, oven and bathroom cleaners which use corrosive chemicals such as **sodium hydroxide** and **sodium hypochlorite** – alias bleach – that can cause severe, sometimes even permanent, burns to eyes and skin.

Look out also, for any products containing **chlorine bleach** and **ammonia** – the highly toxic fumes can at best, be an irritant to any part of your body with which they come into contact, and at worst are likely to react with each other to form **chloramine gases** that are highly damaging to your lungs. Similarly, if chlorine is found alongside acids (most often used in toilet bowl cleaners) then the two will combine to form the very toxic **chlorine gas**. No small wonder that both our general health and the condition of our skin are potentially put at risk every single day of our lives, from these toxic cocktails.

It is important to understand here, as I have mentioned before, that the skin is your body's first line of defense, one of its primary functions being *to protect its inner layers from any nasties thrown at it by the environment.*

Although certain substances are allowed to enter and exit the skin via a process known as **trans-dermal absorption** (an increasingly popular method used in administering nicotine or pain relief patches), the molecular weight of any substance must be very low in order to get past the outer layer or Epidermis. Most of the chemicals you encounter in everyday products however, even if their absorption is blocked by your skin's defense system, will cause problems in many individuals at surface level where they can clog pores, cause extreme irritation and lead to inflammation and the formation of pustules, rashes and the like. These reactions are your skin's response to what it sees as an alien assault on its integrity. On the one hand this would seem to be a good thing, but on the other hand it means that your body is constantly using valuable energy in fighting off this toxic onslaught, that it could more usefully be deploying elsewhere.

Do not forget also, that many products (both household and skincare/cosmetics) come in a spray formulation **which can be inhaled directly into your lungs,** and that almost any toxic substance can gain entry into your bloodstream through broken skin, or through transference to your mouth if you don't wash your hands thoroughly after use.

The Ultimate Guide to Antiaging

Look at the number of chemicals contained in the mouthwash that you happily swirl around your mouth, and maybe even gargle with, no doubt swallowing some in the process. They will pass straight into your blood-stream.

How many times do you shave your armpits with a small hand-held razor, maybe inadvertently cutting your skin, and then use a spray deodorant containing all manner of unpronounceable substances? How often have you slathered sunscreen or after-sun (both full of chemical ingredients) over skin that is blistered and broken from the sun and mosquito bites, leaving the pathways of your body wide open to toxic invasion?

Make-up is another common culprit, as mascara, eye-shadow or eyeliner can so easily be transferred into your eyes, and lipstick (which frequently contains traces of lead) is apparently ingested in pounds over a lifetime of use!

The potential hazards of make-up become very real when you realize that many women wear foundation/concealer/eye shadow/mascara/ lipstick for an average of 12-13 hours a day – more than half of their lifetime! Moreover, a study has revealed that almost 4 out of 10 women frequently leave their make-up on overnight, although whether this is due to vanity or because they simply can't be bothered to take it off is not specified …

… speaking of which, there is currently an issue with cleansing wipes that have become immensely popular with the 21st century woman as a quick and easy way to remove make-up. Sales of these have reportedly more than doubled in the past year. However it is feared that not only are they less than effective at thoroughly cleansing the skin, but that they actually smear make-up across it through the sheer act of wiping. In addition it is very likely that the fluid they contain can cause skin problems such as spots, rashes and the like.

Then of course, there is the big debate over BPA (Bi-Sulphate A), an industrial chemical found in plastics such as water bottles and containers for foods and packaged meals, and in the linings of canned foods such as tinned tomatoes or baked beans. Its critics maintain that it causes a whole load of potential health problems including anxiety and fatigue, specific links to the development of thyroid, lung, breast and prostate cancers, risk of breast cancer, interference with the delicate balance of chemicals in the brain, and hormonal disruption due to the fact that it mimics the effect of oestrogen in your body.

The biggest threat appears to present when plastic is heated, for instance when you microwave food in a plastic container, drink water from a plastic bottle that has heated up in the sun, or put plastic containers in the dishwasher. It is said that the heat generated causes BPA and any other chemicals to seep insidiously into your food, to be ingested.

Ok, we all eat food bought or stored in tins and plastic and as far as I know no-one has ever (directly) died from exposure to BPA through doing this, but how much might it actually contribute towards any of our general health or beauty problems? We often just assume that natural ageing is the cause, or attribute them to poor lifestyle choices such as smoking, drinking or bad nutrition, or just pure bad luck, but **what if** there are other, hidden, contributing factors of which we have not previously been aware?

Some of these body toxins that are absorbed into your system will get stored in fat in order to protect your vital organs (this is a major contributory factor to cellulite but that's another story!). However your body will also eliminate around a third of its accumulated toxins through the surface pores of your skin, where they can contribute to any of the problems mentioned above.

These days more and more people are also finally realizing that the chemicals and synthetic oils used in big brand-name skincare products are bad news for their skin (of which more in Part 2) and there is now a hugely increased demand for natural alternatives. As we have seen, chemicals can be both *harmful to your health and damaging to your skin*, and synthetic oils will *clog your pores and trap toxins inside,* leading to the formation of pimples, blackheads and even rashes over a period of time (one reason why it is such bad practice to leave your make-up on overnight, and why personal hygiene and a good hand-washing technique are essential to avoid cross infection).

This all becomes part of a rather vicious circle in time, as the more damage and trauma caused to the outer layer of your skin the harder it becomes for it to protect itself , therefore allowing even more harmful substances to penetrate it and enter your body. A damaged epidermis also affects your skin's ability to retain moisture, causing dryness which further leads to the formation of fine lines, wrinkles and dull, sagging skin.

The reason that chemicals and other synthetic ingredients are used by so many big manufacturers is - you've guessed it – because *they are cheaper and result in higher profits*. Instead of lining the pockets of these big companies, you should be looking at all the ways you can to naturally improve your diet and lifestyle – together with, if you are still feeling the need to use moisturizer at this point in time, the use of natural plant-based oils that contain lots of nutrients essential to beautiful healthy skin, that are more easily absorbed, and that can help boost your skin's natural properties to tighten and tone from within.

Pesticides and Chemicals in your Food
I think we are all aware of the massive toxic load of pesticides that are to be found in both fresh and processed foods, especially those from supermarkets where the amount of foods showing pesticide residues has more or less doubled in around ten years. A frightening total of 320 pesticides can routinely be used in non-organic farming – the danger

being that we do not know they are there; we cannot see them and so mostly choose to ignore what we don't want to think about.

Fruits are the worst affected with an average of over 90% of produce being contaminated. Grapes have received the worst press, largely due to the fact that the vines are grown year after year in the same soil. This obviously creates a breeding ground for many different types of pests that are routinely annihilated with up to eleven different pesticides, and for this reason the level of contamination in the fruit is often way above the legal limit.

Other fruits at the top of the list include *peaches* and *nectarines, apples*, *strawberries* and *sweet bell peppers*. Most vegetables are also affected, with basic *carrots*, *celery* and *potatoes* being some of the worst offenders. Where vegetables and fruits are not peeled the risk is significantly greater, however if you *do* peel them then you lose a lot of their nutritional content and essential fibre so you really are between the devil and the deep blue sea here. Other foods that commonly contain significant traces of pesticides include *cereal grains* and *flour, cereal bars, dried fruit, bread, crisps* and *rice* – but this list is by no means exhaustive.

To discover the best and worst foods containing pesticides visit the **Pesticide Action Network UK (Pan-uk.org).** Here you will find specific details about the percentage of samples that contain residues, the percentage of samples that contain multiple residues and the percentage of residues that exceed the MRLs (Maximum Recommended Levels).

Those speaking in defense of pesticides will tell us how well they protect the crops and increase production, all of which drives down prices in the increasingly competitive supermarket price-wars. They will also insist that the traces of pesticides in your food are well within acceptably safe limits. However because of the very nature of what they do, pesticides are active against all living organisms and as such pose a very real threat to your health and to the environment in general.

Once again, we need to understand that it is the continual exposure to - and build-up in the system of - these toxic substances that can be harmful. Research has shown that they can result in irritation to the skin, eyes and respiratory system, and potentially cause auto-immune diseases, neurological problems and depression, cancer and birth defects. One of the most common pesticides in regular use (carbendazim) has been found to harm foetal development in the wombs of mammals, and this is present on most fruits, pod beans, spinach and rice. Then of course, there is the devastating effect that pesticides have on the environment, namely soil, water and animal life. But again, that's another story.

I will just make a special mention in this section, of **Soya Beans**. Soya products have long been advertised as a health food, however the beans are in fact full of naturally occurring "anti-nutrients" such as *phytic acid* which can hinder the absorption of vital minerals such as calcium and iron in your body, and can interfere with your body's ability to digest protein. These toxins are normally removed during the process of fermentation (apart from tofu and green edamame beans which are not fermented). However with regard to making soy milk, in addition to the fact that these natural toxins are not guaranteed to be removed, the process adds even more chemicals which are both dangerous and hard to digest so that you end up with a double whammy of harmful ingredients! Non-fermented soy is also very estrogenic and can throw the natural balance of your hormones out of kilter.

Finally, you may have read about the deplorable practices that are involved with most of the meat that you buy on the supermarket shelves and in fast-food outlets, or are unwittingly presented with in institutions like hospitals, schools or anywhere where mass catering on a limited budget leaves the organisers at the mercy of "bulk buying":

- o Most low cost, frozen and processed meats undergo a heinous process that pumps them full of water and nasty chemicals (not at present illegal so long as clearly stated on the nutrition label) under the pretext of enhancing the texture and taste, or making the meat easier to slice.

- o Even sea foods are not exempt, as scallops are routinely soaked in water and phosphates that increase their size and make them look more appealing to consumers, yet remove much of their taste and flavour.

○ The processed ham that you find in your sandwiches is a limp and pithy apology for real meat, having undergone such a destructive process that not only is it choc-full of water and chemical gel but it has almost zero nutritional content. Many consumers don't even notice this appalling lack of taste and texture, especially when the meat is combined with something else strong-tasting like cheese, onion or pickle.

○ However chicken is still, in my opinion, one of the worst examples of "meddling with nature" that I have come across, with some imported, frozen chicken breasts being actually thawed out and plumped up with water and chemicals before being *re-frozen* and sold in many of our leading supermarkets. Some chicken breasts contain a staggering 20% of water - no doubt those belonging to poor little battery farmed chickens that never see the light of day, are fed an unnatural and highly processed diet and do not have space to develop and grow.

How can any meat from such a source be good for you? Why contaminate your body with what is at best a mockery of real food? Water obviously, is a much cheaper commodity than meat and this is why it is so attractive to suppliers and retailers, who can then charge consumers over the odds for what appears to be a succulent bargain but is in fact a sub-standard and potentially harmful piece of produce.

The problem is, we don't eat "whole" food anymore – we eat mass-produced "food-like" products. At the end of the day, all these unnatural and inflammatory substances that we find in our foods, together with other risk factors such as smoking and alcohol, put the liver under great strain and affect its innate ability to repair itself. This can lead to liver damage, and ultimately cancer – and as we have seen, any illness will potentially have a major impact upon ageing and the health and appearance of your skin.

Air Pollution, for example smog, traffic fumes, smoke and industrial waste is a significant enemy of your skin, and can cause premature ageing particularly on the more exposed face, neck and hands. It does this by drawing oxygen out of the skin's cells (as we have seen, one of the leading causes of ageing), increasing free radicals and the effect of UV radiation, and hastening the breakdown of elastin fibres.

Air pollution has adverse effects on the appearance and texture of your skin which, if subjected to long-term exposure to high level pollutants, may eventually become dull and lack-lustre, with clogged pores, a lack of vitality and the possible development of spots, blemishes and fine lines. The first thing many people do in response is to reach for an expensive face-cream that promises the earth but actually, even if the active ingredients were to manage to penetrate your skin's barrier, does nothing to address the root cause. Fact!

Furthermore, contaminants in the atmosphere can interfere with your skin's ability to regulate moisture levels, and some people may even develop allergies, skin disease or pigmentation problems.

As you will by now realize, these problems with your skin once again stem from an issue related to your general health, the root cause in this instance being the potentially decreased ability of the lungs to get sufficient oxygen into your body due to intense irritation, and the increased production of mucus in the airways which will narrow in response. This poses a particularly high risk area for anybody who regularly exercises outside in urban areas, such as runners, cyclists, power-walkers, dog walkers etc - and anyone who suffers from a chronic lung disease such as emphysema, asthma or bronchitis could find their conditions worsening as a result of air contaminants.

The main dangers lie in three areas: *ozone levels*, *fine particles* in the atmosphere, and *carbon monoxide*:

- **Ozone** – aka smog – is formed when sunlight reacts with traffic fumes, and continued prolonged exposure can narrow the airways in your lungs, making it harder for oxygen exchange to take place. It is at its worst when the sun is at its peak, and can cause breathing to become more laboured and stressful over time.

○ **Fine particles** are deposited directly into the atmosphere by traffic fumes or from industrial sources, and can cause irritation, inflammation, stress and an increased production of mucus in the airways deep within your lungs. The tiniest particles (invisible to the naked eye) can even find their way into the bloodstream.

○ Finally, **Carbon Monoxide**, present in cigarette smoke and exhaust fumes, significantly reduces, and even prevents, the uptake of oxygen by the blood.

If you are young and in good health, you are unlikely to notice any short-term effects from air pollution but as with any toxic substances the long-term effects can be devastating in later life. *In fact air pollution is said to be responsible for an almost unbelievable 29,000 premature deaths a year in the UK.*

Another potential danger that many people are unaware of is the concentration of air pollutants in the home which, in the confines of a restricted space, can actually be considerably higher than that outside. The main culprits are cigarette smoke, dust and dust-mite droppings, pollen from indoor flowers, moulds, fumes from wood burners, heaters, boilers etc. and a host of household products (as discussed in the previous section) that contain VOCs (volatile organic compounds) which can remain in your home not only for days but for years. Varnishes and paints are some of the worst offenders here, as even if the lids are firmly in place they can still emit potentially dangerous fumes. See Section 3 for ways in which you can reduce your exposure to indoor and outdoor air pollution.

Weight Loss may do wonders for your appearance and your self-esteem, but random or faddy dieting is not good news for your skin. We have already discussed the effects of low fat diets, and how these inevitably lead to us consuming more sugar, the excess of which is then converted into "bad" fat in your body. We have also seen how a certain amount of the right sort of fat is vital to preserve the health and radiance of your skin.

Dieting is also bad for your skin in that, by cutting out various foodstuffs from your diet, you run the risk of becoming deficient in one or more nutrients that your skin so badly needs to keep it looking young and healthy.

Also if your weight loss is too quick, then it will cause your skin to become saggy and wrinkly over your new, thinner frame – and trust me, this is not a good look.

There are many reasons why a person may put on weight, such as eating the wrong type of food, insufficient exercise, over-eating through stress, limited movement due to chronic pain, certain medications and pregnancy. In each case it is the **rate** and **severity** of the weight loss that determines the success (or otherwise) of the skin's natural elasticity in preventing sagging and stretch marks.

The skin has a wonderful ability to adapt to moderate fluctuations in body weight, but fast, extreme or continual weight loss (yo-yo dieting) challenges this ability to the utmost, often resulting in folds of loose, defeated skin that can no longer repair itself and that has lost its strength and tone (I am talking in particular here about the body, as facial and neck skin does not react as drastically due to the fact that comparatively little excess weight is stored in these parts). So be warned, if you are thinking of going on a diet, *slow and gradual weight loss is the only way forward if you want to preserve your skin's elasticity and tone*.

Lack of Exercise: Exercise increases blood flow, thereby improving circulation by carrying oxygen and nutrients to the working cells throughout your body, including to your skin. As we have seen, blood flow has a further vital role in that it helps remove waste products, including free radicals, from these cells.

Regular exercise also has the effect of decreasing the number of stress hormones such as cortisol in your body, and stimulating the release of your body's "feel good" chemicals, called *endorphins*, from your brain. The ensuing decrease in stress, apart from promoting relaxed and healthy skin in general, can be beneficial in the long term to some skin conditions such as acne, eczema, rosacea and psoriasis. Research indicates that the oil-producing sebaceous glands in your skin are stimulated by stress hormones, thus resulting in an over-production of oil which further exacerbates these conditions.

Just to make you aware, if you have problem skin and exercise *too* strenuously, you can experience short-term flare ups caused by salt from perspiration - in which case you should take advice from your specialist on the best way to combat this. Again it is all about balance.

So now you are more aware of the benefits of exercise for your skin, you will be able to understand how a lack of it, especially in combination with any other bad practice such as smoking, alcohol or a poor diet, will be most detrimental both in the short and long- term.

STRESS: It is a well known fact that stress can cause skin problems in many individuals something that scientists call Psycho Dermatology. Your mind and your body interact extremely closely, and the physiological reaction of your body to stress prompts an increased level of secretion of **cortisol** from your adrenal glands. Cortisol is a steroid, and is also one of the primary stress hormones released during your body's primitive "fight or flight" response to stress. It stimulates the release of glucose, fats and amino

acids into the bloodstream to meet the demand for fast energy.

An unfortunate by-product of this process is inflammation in your body's organs including your skin, also there may be an increase in your skin's oil production, both of which risk making you more prone to pimples, spots, rashes, itchiness and dryness. It is for this reason that many existing skin complaints such as acne, eczema, psoriasis, rosacea and hives, are frequently made worse by stress, which is a well known trigger.

Stress can also cause or exacerbate problems with your blood pressure (which may become raised), your respiratory system (through panic attacks and hyperventilation), your heart rate (may become rapid) and your digestive and immune systems (which may become sluggish and inefficient).

This assault on your bodily systems can result in any of the following: tension; insomnia and headaches; irritability; anger; inability to concentrate; acute anxiety or depression; loss of sex drive and loss of vitality. Additionally stress has been identified as a cause of infertility.

Stress becomes doubly harmful once people start looking for ways to relieve it. Very frequently they may turn to alcohol, smoking or drugs, which instead of relaxing the body serve only to keep it in a stressed state.

Other unhealthy ways of dealing with stress include not wanting to get out of bed in the mornings, crying a lot, nail-biting, withdrawing from friends, family and activities, becoming a "couch potato" in front of the television or computer screen, and venting all that pent-up anger or frustration on other people. These same individuals will be extremely likely to neglect their skin, as their level of stress prevents them from maintaining a daily routine or even, in some cases, not caring about what they look like at all.

A study way back in 2004 discovered an important link between a healthy, stress-free lifestyle and the ageing process: Within the cells of your body are **chromosomes**, and each chromosome has a tiny "cap" of DNA called a **telomere** on the end (rather like a small knot at the end of a length of cotton) which prevents deterioration and protects the lifespan of the cell containing it.

It was already a known fact that telomeres become naturally shorter with age, but what the study found out was that those individuals who had endured long-term psychological stress had prematurely ageing cells and carried a higher risk of increasing health problems and an earlier death.

I should also mention here that anything that causes direct trauma to the skin itself, such as injury, extreme heat or cold, tight clothing, insect bites, exposure to chemicals or other irritants, sun exposure and tattoos, results in the skin being in a state of stress that can cause problems both in the short and long term.

Apart from the fact that tattoos can stretch and horribly distort the skin, many of the inks used have been linked to cancer-causing chemicals that can easily get into the bloodstream and reach the body's internal organs. They have also been shown to cause irreversible damage to collagen tissue.

And of course wherever the surface of the skin is broken it is a source of both great traumatic stress and potential infection. Remember that *your skin sits better over relaxed muscles, and is therefore less likely to wrinkle*!

Lack of Sleep: Although lack of sleep can commonly be a by-product (cause or effect) of stress, I have dealt with it separately as there are many other causes to consider such as illness, pain or discomfort, sleep disorders, lifestyle, shift work, an over-active mind, a new baby in the household - you get the picture …

While chronic sleep deprivation has long been recognized as having major links to many serious medical conditions, its effect upon skin ageing has only recently become a subject of interest and research. It is now claimed that lack of - or poor quality - sleep can as much as double the signs of skin ageing, as it causes a state of stress within the body. It can also weaken the skin's ability to rejuvenate and repair itself at night and to recover from sun damage.

Working night shifts is a prime example of how the body's genetic make-up is thrown into complete disarray as a result of unnatural sleep patterns, resulting in a state of chaos deep within our DNA and laying our body's pathways wide open to long-term health problems and ageing issues.

In a US study commissioned by a leading skincare company, 60 pre-menopausal women between the ages of 30 and 49 (exactly half of whom suffered from poor or insufficient sleep), were involved in tests to measure the degree of moisture loss in the skin. Those with poor quality sleep were found to have twice as much moisture loss as the good sleepers and their skin showed significantly more signs of ageing in terms of poor colour, lack of elasticity and an increased number of fine lines. This is the first time that poor sleep quality has been scientifically proven both to accelerate signs of ageing in the skin and to weaken the ability of the skin to repair itself at night (the time when skin detoxification is most active).

Chronic Pain is that which is present for a long period of time and is either resistant to medication and other treatments, or needs constant treatment at home or in hospital in order to keep it at a manageable level. Some examples of chronic pain include arthritis, back pain, migraines/tension headaches, burns, vasculitis (which translates as inflammation of the blood vessels), inflammatory bowel disease, cancer, sports injuries and neuropathic pain. A person can suffer simultaneously

from two or more chronic pain conditions which can be extremely debilitating.

Different conditions can affect the skin in different ways. For example when someone is in pain their muscles are tight and in a state of tension, and this can restrict blood flow in that area. This could result in a change in colour and texture of the surrounding skin.

Neuropathic pain such as sciatica, neuralgia and diabetic neuropathy can also cause these changes, and most probably alter the way certain sensations are felt such as touch and temperature. This results from damage to the peripheral ("near the surface") nerves and to those outside the spinal cord and brain that service the internal organs, muscles and the skin. When a person is near death one of the first warning signs is the look of their skin, which becomes colourless and like parchment due to the shut-down of all the bodily systems and the cessation of life-giving blood flow to the body's organs and the skin.

Whatever the type of pain however, it can potentially or actually cause lack of sleep, stress, loss of appetite (leading to inadequate nutrition and weight *loss*), comfort eating (which combined with restricted mobility may result in weight *gain*) and a blitz of toxins and chemicals from various medications, all of which spell suicide for the skin. Substances such as *phthalates*, *heavy metals* and *commercial preservatives* used to coat and to preserve billions of over-the-counter medications, are chemically toxic and can disrupt the normal functioning of the hormonal system, also recent research has shown that anti-inflammatory drugs such as Ibuprofen and Diclofenac can cause an irregular heartbeat that may increase the risk of a stroke.

The same is true of prescription drugs. *Chemotherapy and radiation,* for example, can both severely compromise the outer layer of your skin by interfering with cell renewal (which, if you remember, takes place in the epidermis) causing extreme dryness, irritation, rashes and thin, fragile skin that is easily damaged.

Diuretics (prescribed to rid your body of excess fluid) can also cause dryness by very virtue of the fact that they remove water from your body and therefore potentially also from your skin during long-term use, or if the balance of medication is wrong. The problematic "pooling" of fluid, most commonly seen in the ankles and lower legs and called **oedema**, is a by-product of certain medical conditions such as heart failure, alcoholic liver cirrhosis, hepatitis and coeliac disease. It can also be caused through pregnancy, trauma, obesity and/or prolonged inactivity.

Every one of these conditions has the potential to cause long or short-term problems for your skin but this is just one example where the treatment itself is almost equally as damning as the condition it is attempting to control.

All of the above highlights the indisputable connection between your skin and your overall health, further proving that the key to ageless, beautiful skin is to do everything you can to keep your body in tip top condition inside and out.

Sun Exposure: I have deliberately left sun exposure until last, as I actually believe that – with proper care – sunlight is not only good but essential for us and for our skin, despite the bad press it has received. There are critics who believe that getting a tan is a sign of skin damage from the sun's rays. I myself cannot see how a gradual, light tan can be deemed to be unhealthy when it is actually *the body's natural defense against sun damage.* A build-up of melanin (the pigment produced by the melanocytes in your epidermis) helps block UV rays and also serves as a powerful anti-oxidant.

The Case *for ...*

Sunlight is so good for our psychological and physical states. It activates a gene which enhances our sex drive, it releases endorphins (our happiness hormones), and also leptin which helps burn fat to keep us slim. Recent research suggests that it also lowers blood pressure which in turn reduces the risk of heart attacks and strokes, and that it can protect against breast cancer. Most importantly sunlight is the main source of vitamin D, the "sunshine vitamin", lack of which can cause a serious health problem by blocking the body's absorption of calcium and phosphorus.

Vitamin D deficiency is an increasingly common condition, especially in children, that doctors are only more recently becoming aware of since it was eradicated after the Second World War. It can result in chronic mineral imbalance, extreme fatigue and depression, severe cognitive impairment and bone deterioration. It has also been linked to multiple sclerosis. Vitamin D deficiency has reared its ugly head even more so since the advocates of safe tanning began warning us of the dreadful consequences of being out in the sun, and how we should use a Factor 25 at the very least in order to protect from skin cancer.

Only recently I read an article in one of the daily papers about a six year old boy who has developed rickets caused by a lack of vitamin D. His mother had been slathering a Factor 50 sunscreen over him every time he went out to play, believing she was doing the right thing and protecting him from skin cancer. Instead he was found to have a serious vitamin D deficiency which had lead to rickets, a very painful, bone-softening disease which may leave him with permanent damage.

○ Vitamin D deficiency has increased four-fold over the last decade as children spend more and more time indoors in front of the television or playing with computer games, while the current obsession with low-fat foods and ready meals compromises the quality of their diet. As children, we were given daily cod-liver oil, introduced by the Government during the Second World War to combat this disease. We played outside, took part in out-of-door activities and we ate whole, full-fat food that was mostly home-cooked.

○ As a result of these measures, rickets became a disease of the past. It is due entirely to current lifestyle trends - namely poor diet and our aversion to sunlight – fuelled by media hype, that it is on the rise again.

The Case *against*

However, lack of understanding and respect for the sun's rays can indeed cause untold damage, particularly to fair or sensitive skin. How many times do you see holidaymakers after their first day on the beach, unattractive in fiery lobster red after hours of sun exposure with inadequate protection or cover-up – ugly strap marks showing, skin already peeling. Make no mistake about it, *this can seriously and irreparably damage the structure of your skin*, causing it at best to develop premature lines and wrinkles, and at worst to develop serious conditions such as skin cancer.

Yes, if genetically you have the type of skin that will tolerate the sun and that tans easily, then you are lucky as a gradually acquired suntan provides natural protection against UV rays. *But* a red, burnt and blistered skin is a direct result of sun damage and not only is this grossly unattractive but also highly dangerous. In addition to the very obvious risk of skin cancer it will damage the elastin fibres in the skin, causing it to lose its firmness and elasticity and further speeding up the effects of ageing. Not only that, but in stripping the skin of vitamin A, sun damage will also rob it of its innate ability to repair damage and to boost collagen production.

Flaky, peeling skin is a warning sign that you have tanned too quickly and allowed your skin to dry out through over-exposure and the wrong sunscreen for your skin type. It also suggests that your skin was radically dry and not in peak condition to begin with. Relaxed, well-nourished and well-hydrated skin will not peel, something that those who are used to - or live in – a hot climate are well aware of. So if you don't want to look like a tourist, or someone unused to the sun, take sensible precautions and acquire your tan nice and slowly!

Something else to be aware of as you become older is that in middle life your oestrogen production will start to decrease and the balance of bacteria and fungi naturally existing on your skin may change. Again this process will happen sooner in life for some than for others. Exposure to strong sunlight (along with drinking alcohol and eating spicy foods) will actually react with the process and make it worse, causing skin complaints such as rosacea, a condition that presents with flushing, broken veins and pus spots.

Above all remember the drying effect of sun and wind upon your skin, and at the risk of sounding repetitious I will say again in conclusion:

"Wherever the skin is dry wrinkles will eventually appear"

In addition, therefore, to protecting your skin on the outside it is vital to keep fully hydrated from the inside by drinking plenty of water.

"Hydration, Hydration, Hydration!"

This is so, so important.

Read the corresponding section in Part 2 to find out how you can naturally protect your skin without the use of potentially damaging commercial sunscreens.

Summary

You have now reached the end of Part 1 of "The Ultimate Guide to Antiaging" so well done for persevering this far! I hope you feel that you have learnt something really valuable, and have a far greater insight into what makes your skin "tick", why **the only way** to restore and/or preserve your youthful looks and beautiful skin or to find the ultimate solution for skin problems, is by using an internal health approach focusing on lifestyle and diet.

Go back and read Part 1 again – it all adds up, doesn't it? It makes sense, there is no other solution that will give you such naturally, beautiful and long-term results *"without the price-tag, without the pain, and without any hidden nasties such as parabens that can dry or irritate your skin...*the **One** *amazingly simple and natural solution that keeps your skin radiant and glowing from top to toe (yes, your whole body and not just your face) and also helps problem skin - a strategy that delivers sensational results every time* BECAUSE *it works!"* You have now done most of the ground work, so "Congratulations" - you are almost ready to take start taking action!

Still to come in Part 2: **Irresistible** advertising by large cosmetic companies and how it preys on our vanity and our emotions. **How** chemicals used in anti-freeze and oven cleaner are turning up in organic skin creams. **Why** some moisturizers may actually *increase* the signs of ageing. **Why** you should never waste money on creams containing collagen and elastin – and lots more! Finally then, I'll be telling you in detail exactly what you need to do (or not, as the case may be!) to future-proof your skin and turn that ageing process belly-up!

Ready to go? Then read on ...

Section Two: the Myth, the Lies and the Truth

Chapter One

WHY do we fall for it? The sneaky secrets of the advertising world revealed

We are bombarded with advertising every day of our lives through radio and television commercials, magazines and newspapers, web-site ads and emails, billboards, posters, flyers, ads on the back of buses ... I'm sure you can think of more, the list just goes on and on - and it all has one unwavering aim which is *to persuade us to buy something*, be it a product, service or an amenity.

Two things are identified when creating a product for sale: a) **The Problem**, and b) **The Solution**. Marry the two together with ingenious advertising and you create **Desire**. That is the simple formula used by almost every company on the planet, to make their money!

Advertising can be clever, sophisticated, manipulative, cunning and persuasive. Companies pay a fortune for the services of professional copy writers who know exactly which buttons to press to create that all-consuming feeling of desire – "powerful" words and phrases that will have us reaching for our wallet even quicker than our sense of reason deserts us!

Nowadays advertising is targeted more selectively to a "niche" market rather than indiscriminately to the masses, particularly in magazines and on the internet. Ads for weight loss will be placed on niche websites and in magazines like Weight Watchers or Slimming World ... ads for beauty products in the health & beauty niche on the internet or in women's magazines, etc.

By doing this, companies are advertising solely to those consumers very likely to have an interest in their products. This makes much more sense from their point of view as, apart from generating a far greater response, it is also more cost effective. It does however mean that as a consumer, every time you buy a magazine in, say, the health and beauty niche, you will be bombarded by page after page of adverts all targeted specifically to this market. Some people quite enjoy browsing through these ads, but they can be a source of irritation to others who feel that they detract from the value of the magazine.

In the beauty industry advertising is aimed at women wanting to improve their appearance and self image, to be attractive to the opposite sex and to slow down the signs of ageing. It preys on the fact that most women have an inferiority complex about their looks, an inbuilt desire to look like the images of models in the ads. They aspire to *be* them. In fact the beauty industry is constantly being accused of using unrealistic and unachievable images in order to highlight what women consider to be their bad points and thereby lowering their confidence and self esteem. The expectation is, of course, that they will then buy the advertised product in order to solve whatever problem it is they think they have.

Our idea of beauty has been so distorted by visions of stick-thin models and airbrushed photos of impossibly long-limbed and flawlessly tanned women with not a visible wrinkle in sight, that our antennae are already quivering on red alert by the time the next anti-ageing ad hits the media, full of seductive promise …

… because what we are actually buying here is **the promise** … the promise of youth, confidence and beauty sitting so tantalizingly in that little jar of mysterious magic wherein lies the key, the overnight solution (because most of us are basically lazy and do not want to put any effort in!) to all our problems, the promise that we too can look *like the girl in that ad*. We imagine the luxuriant texture of the cream, the sensual feel of it on our skin, the magical transformation reflected to us in the mirror the next morning after it has worked its overnight magic. And the smaller the jar and the higher the price tag, the greater is our perception of the credibility and the worth of this product we so desire.

It's a bit like buying a lottery ticket in that you don't pay £1-2 for just a piece of paper with six numbers printed on it, you are buying the promise of what those numbers would mean to you and your family if they were to win, how they would change your life forever. If your numbers don't come up of course, as usually happens, then the piece of paper gets scrumpled up and thrown away. It no longer has any value, rather like the latest anti-wrinkle cream gathering dust on your bathroom shelf because it has failed to live up to expectations, expectations born out of headlines such as "**Miracle cream holds the key to eternal youth**"; "**New anti-wrinkle serum, sold out on day one**" or "**Instant Facelift in a tube – 10.000 sold in 48 hours**".

Call me a cynic but in my opinion this is less about problem solving than about persuading as many people as possible to spend as much money as possible and as often as possible, by creating a "buzz" around the product, a buying frenzy. And we fall for it time and time again.

I can think of no better way to conclude this chapter than to repeat the words I used way back in the Introduction to this book: "Clever advertising is all about desire. We see something, we want it. We may not need it, but because of the compelling nature of the ad we overwhelmingly DESIRE it, we are afraid of missing out, we HAVE to have it".

The End!

Chapter Two

The Frightening Truth about Botox and Cosmetic Surgery

Everything you have just read in the preceding chapter can also be applied to the advertising hype for cosmetic surgery, botox, fillers and the like, only an even greater price tag and potentially a lot of pain and discomfort is involved before we reap the promised reward. But desperation, like love, is blind, which is why this industry continues to grow and prosper through a failing economy.

Take **botox**, for example: at around £150 a pop (some clinics can charge twice this amount) it is not cheap, and the effects are only temporary. It needs repeating every six months or so in order to preserve "the look".

It is worrying to realize that supposedly reputable consultants are actively encouraging young twenty-something women to have botox on the grounds that it's better to start young before their wrinkles and crow's feet (two of the major concerns) take hold. Worrying too, that botox is becoming somewhat of a cult with this age-group, almost a status symbol in fact. They are obsessed with their appearance and with the idea of age prevention, an obsession fuelled largely by the media and in particular by TV programs such as "The Only Way Is Essex". In some cases having botox has become just a matter of course; as commonplace as popping in for a facial after work with your friends - and really no big deal.

Now if it was even just a matter of the cost it would be bad enough, but think on this: Apart from having the potential to cause pain and discomfort botox can cause very discomfiting side effects, namely localized redness, tenderness, inflammation and swelling at the injection site and, even worse, drooping eyelids or eyebrows, as a result of *muscle atrophy*.

Muscle atrophy is something that happens when muscles are not used for a period of time (as happens when you have botox) and begin to waste away. Of course the effect of this is going to be far more noticeable in younger people who still have a naturally good muscle tone, and the effect can be extremely ageing. This is ironic, as people having botox believe that they are turning back the clock whereas in fact they can potentially end up by making themselves look even older. Those who are addicted may even find that they eventually become immune to the treatments, which would then no longer work - at which point the reversal of their skin to its previous state would be drastically more noticeable by comparison.

So, taking all these facts into consideration, botox is at best a mostly unnecessary waste of money, and at worst an unspeakably traumatic experience for your skin. It is horrifying to realize that there are people giving botox literally in their back yard, and who, due to the current lack of legislation (now under review), are not medical professionals and offer no mention of any qualifications.

At the most basic level, when you inject anyone for any reason there is always a risk of infection, so imagine the potential of what could go wrong in this kind of situation. I read only recently about a woman who, having passed herself off as a highly qualified beautician, was charging what her customers thought was a bargain price of £90 per session for cheap Botox bought off the internet. In fact her credentials were false and her deception was only brought to light when a client experienced a bad reaction.

Cosmetic surgery is an even worse case scenario, as whatever you are told the results cannot be guaranteed and the risks are far, far greater.

There are currently plans to bring in new guidelines for those undergoing cosmetic procedures, which hopefully will give the consumer more redress if things go wrong and will also ensure that only medically qualified professionals can inject cosmetic fillers into patients'/clients' faces. However it is feared that even if these measures become law, it won't be enough to stop cowboy surgeons.

Remember that, even if the operation is a success in the sense that you don't end up with dreadful scarring or worse, you will not necessarily look any younger - or even better – for the amount of money, pain and discomfort invested. Some of these procedures can radically change the way you look, and if you were not born that way then this new image may not be right for you, and may even appear comical.

It is sad that so many women have such a poor perception of themselves, and feel under so much pressure to look good. Cosmetic surgery in effect, becomes a shield behind which to hide from a deeper and more pressing psychological problem. It is, up to a point, more understandable with those in the public eye - particularly in professions such as TV presenting and acting where the pressure is on to compete with younger women for the best jobs.

In the States, cosmetic surgery is the norm with most actresses of around 30, but it is also far from uncommon in the UK. Celebrities such as the actress Leslie Ash, and the glamour girl/actress Alicia Duvall immediately spring to mind. Alicia Duvall has reportedly suffered from body dysmorphic disorder, and has undergone over 100 operations at a total cost of around £1.5million. Despite the astronomical cost she admits to having residual pain and discomfort, and that her face feels immobile from the effects of so much surgery (one very good reason, I would have thought, why this would not be a good idea for any actress who needs to use facial expression as a means to portraying her screen/stage character).

Unfortunately cosmetic surgery is like decorating, you have one thing done and it immediately shows up some-thing else, some other "flaw" that "needs correcting". It is almost impossible to draw a line. It becomes an obsession, a lifetime's commitment. And for what? Stretched, shiny skin over a face that now has no character or expression? Unnaturally full, pouting lips that fail to marry up with the rest of your features? Breast implants that eventually cause all sorts of problems where before there were none? Having the face of a 25 year old but the neck/décolletage/stomach/hands/feet etc. of someone who's fifty?

The only excuse I can find for cosmetic procedures is where there is a problem that may adversely affect a person's health or mental state and even then I would say proceed with extreme caution.

I would far rather see women who age naturally and beautifully, who exude character, are fun-loving and squeeze every last drop out of life, because these individuals attract others to them like a magnet, they have an aura that makes people want to be around them. And THAT, when combined with a radiant, healthy skin from the kind of internal health approach that I am recommending, is what constitutes true beauty. After all, your face is the sum total not only of your genetic heritage but of your life's experiences – and you should wear it with pride!

Chapter Three

You won't believe they put *THIS* in your skincare products

These days it is a widely accepted fact that we do not know what's in the food we eat, and even when listed on the labels of packaged and processed foods it is usually easier to ignore what we can't pronounce or what is not immediately recognizable as an ingredient.

The same is unfortunately true of the majority of skincare products, sadly even some of those listed as being organic. Nothing is sacred - it is yet another example of big brand companies putting profit before ethics, and while some of these companies do actually seem to be making an effort to update their products and remove certain of the offending chemicals from their formulations, others are still insisting that the levels of preservative they use fall well within the guidelines approved by the European Commission and that as such their products are safe for consumer use.

In Part 1 I talked at some length, it being quite a weighty topic, about the general effects of chemicals and toxins in your body and on your skin. In this chapter I am focusing specifically on a certain chemical that has had a huge amount of publicity in recent months, and that has apparently triggered one of the most significant skin allergy epidemics in history. In fact the evidence against this chemical is so strong that, at the time of writing, the European Commission is taking steps to ban it from all leave-on cosmetics, and to drastically reduce its concentration in rinse-off products such as shampoos and shower gels – despite many companies strongly denying that it causes any harm.

It is its current bad press that has prompted me to focus on this chemical in particular, as being a blatant example of the appallingly toxic substances that skincare companies have been adding to products that we routinely apply to, and leave on, our skin.

And even if, by the time you read this, this particular offender has indeed been subject to a partial ban then let it be a reminder of the many others that still have approval for use, and that therefore continue to pose a threat to your health and to the condition of your skin.

The name of this chemical is **methylisothiazolinone** (**MI**), and it is a synthetic chemical preservative designed to extend the shelf life of a product and/or to prevent it from deteriorating.

It is found in a large number of house-hold items such as paint, cleaning products, air fresheners, and washing up liquid. *It is also used in engine oil and anti-freeze*. And it is this same chemical that is added to a large majority of products you put on your skin! Personally I have come across it mostly in hair care products I have used, but it is also to be found in shower and bath creams/gels, moisturizers, sun screens, personal wipes, liquid soap, make up ... the list goes on and on.

Next time you find yourself in Boots, Superdrug or the like, spend a few minutes browsing the shelves and see just how many products you can find that contain this chemical in their list of ingredients (clue: these are companies that are both household names and trusted brands!).

Many years ago MI was used in conjunction with another preservative by the name of **methylchloroisothiazolinone** (**MCI**) until a wave of allergic skin reactions prompted some adjustments in the level of permitted concentrations.

The upshot of this period of testing (which lasted for over ten years) was that MCI was deemed to be the most likely cause of all the problems - and so from 2005 MI was approved by the European Commission as a preservative able to be used in its own right in skincare and cosmetic products, and at a higher concentration than previously. Because it was assumed to be safe at that time, and consumers weren't routinely patch tested for allergic reactions, it wasn't until four years later that the existence of a potentially serious problem was acknowledged.

Data gathered from patch centers across the UK indicated that up to 10% of people were allergic to both MCI *and* MI – way above the usually predicted 1-2% for any given product and as such completely unacceptable.

Dermatologists believe that the scale of the problem is due in part to the fact that so many millions of people are now using products that contain the chemicals, but also because continued exposure to even a relatively low concentration of toxins will have a cumulative effect in the system, building up into proportions that will contribute to major problems with health in the long-term.

Both MI and MCI (for the latter is still popping up in skincare products despite its previous bad press) can cause a battalion of symptoms in susceptible individuals: rashes, redness and swelling (particularly around the face), itching, lumps and blisters, scaling skin, in fact all the symptoms that you may expect from an allergic reaction. Hair care products specifically, can result in eczema around the hairline and eyelids.

Symptoms are generally localized to begin with (they appear in the area where the product was first applied) but may then spread to other adjacent areas, and a reactive response can take up to 24 hours to present with symptoms. It is generally agreed that the chemicals have absolutely no benefit in any product that is left on the skin and in fact experts have suggested that they could even, in some cases, cause cancer or nerve damage.

Now when you consider that MI is **just one** of the myriad of ingredients (mostly unpronounceable) to be found in trusted products that you use every day of your life, it poses the very real question, "Can your face cream actually be doing more harm than good to your skin?"

The thing I find unforgivable is that several of the big brand beauty products labeled and advertised as organic, have also been found to contain traces of these toxic chemicals. Unfortunately there are no existing laws to regulate the labeling of organic beauty products (unlike organic foods) although there are in existence self-certification schemes run by voluntary organizations such as **The Soil Association**. In order to qualify, companies have to meet certain criteria which include banning any stipulated chemicals from their products and being able to certify that they only use plant based and organically grown ingredients.

All this bad press simply reinforces my argument that an internal health approach is not only the best but the safest and by far the cheapest way to guarantee healthy and beautiful skin in the long term. The general rule of thumb is this: *If you can't pronounce it or you wouldn't eat it then don't put it on your skin* and most certainly – in the case of what you eat – *don't let it past your lips!*

Chapter Four

The number one reason why you should *never* waste money on creams containing collagen and elastin - skincare companies will *not* want you to know this …

Having read and become familiar with the structure and function of your skin as explained in Part 1 of this book, you will remember that one of the main functions of the outer layer of your skin is *to protect its inner layers from any "nasties" thrown at it by the environment",* to resist and reject any unrecognized substances that try to penetrate its surface. It is basically the first-line defense system in place to protect your body.

You may also remember that two of the most vital components of your skin, collagen and elastin – so crucial to preserving your skin's integrity and elasticity and therefore of the utmost relevance to the whole anti-ageing issue – are only to be found buried deep in the dermis or middle layer of your skin. The major problem for beauty/skin care experts therefore, has been to try to find a viable method of transporting the molecules of collagen and elastin contained in their products, to that part of the skin where they are needed.

At the time of writing, this problem has not been overcome satisfactorily because:

a. the molecules are consistently too large to pass through the skin's barrier so mostly just sit helplessly on the surface until washed away

b. even were they able to reach the skin's deeper layers, the amounts used are far too small and/or in the wrong proportions, to make any significant difference (this is in no small part down to the expense of the said ingredients, IF good quality collagen is used which, unfortunately, is not very often the case) and

c. *were they actually to have the ability to penetrate the skin and enter the bloodstream then the product would need to be re-classified as a medicine.*

One of the ways in which skincare companies have attempted to solve this apparently insurmountable problem is to use tiny synthetic vesicles made out of the same phospholipids as a cell membrane, to act as transporters for their anti-ageing compounds. However research has shown that, far from transporting molecules of collagen and elastin deep into the skin, these liposomes break up more or less on contact with its surface, which pretty much negates all the fancy claims made about their efficacy!

Most consumers know that the natural depletion of collagen and elastin in their skin plays a major part in the development of wrinkles and contribution to ageing. Advertisers have made sure of this with a lot of inflated hype about their products over the years, and of course there has been a lot of related coverage in the media, particularly women's and health and beauty magazines and the national press.

What consumers are patently **not** clear about is the amount of absorption of these various products into that part of their skin where they can actually do any good. Clever advertising and extreme care over the wording of any claims made by skincare companies mean that women are successfully being conned into paying a high price for products that do not, and in point of fact **cannot**, deliver. Quite simply, the mere mention of collagen guarantees that a product will fly off the shelves, and what the beauty industry relies upon quite heavily is *lack of background knowledge* on the part of the consumer, coupled with *fear* (of looking older) and a *desire* to regain the smooth and beautiful skin of their youth.

Do not for one minute, imagine that these companies care about you personally. They don't. However you *are* important to them in that you have the potential to make them rich – and therein lies the truth of the matter.

The most that these products (like *any* skin cream) can do is to smooth and moisturize the cells on the surface of your epidermis to give a temporary look of brightness and a nice, soft velvety feel to the touch – and I am not disputing that this is something they can achieve very satisfactorily.

However as your skin's surface cells are being constantly shed and replaced by new ones, and as the major ingredients in these products are incapable of penetrating further than the skin's surface, then it isn't hard to understand that any such effect can only be a very temporary one and certainly not enough to justify either the price or the expectations invested.

So I will say it again: *the only way that you can effect a viable and long-term change in your skin is through committing to an internal health approach that addresses all the issues - dehydration, poor nutrition, poor circulation, inflammation and free radical formation – which are the **root cause** of all your health and beauty issues.*

Chapter Five

So is it really necessary to use a moisturiser at all? The answer – and the reasoning behind it – may surprise you

Well, as women apparently spend around £550 million a year on the stuff, then it would appear that most of us regard it as something we can't live without. However recent conjecture by some experts suggests that long-term use of moisturiser can actually have the adverse effect of making the skin drier. The principle behind this is one that, as a nurse, I find easy to understand and to accept. If you remember I touched upon it earlier when talking about the structure of the epidermis: *"Once we start interfering with the natural processes in our bodies, our bodies will become lazy and less efficient in response. If you slather moisturiser onto your skin day in, day out, then your body will register this and eventually see no further need to continue producing its own natural oils"*.

This idea that interfering with the natural mechanism of our body causes it to become lazy and inefficient (in that particular area in which we have "interfered") is a well known concept in the medical world …

An example is *Hypothyroidism*, a condition in which a patient has low levels of thyroxin and needs a daily "top-up" in the form of medication. The dose has to be very carefully balanced for that patient's individual needs, because if too much is given their body will be fooled into thinking that there is no longer a problem. The result of this is that it will stop making the effort to produce even the small amount of thyroxin that it was struggling to produce before and the patient will end up needing even larger doses to compensate.

The same principal applies to your skin. It is indeed true that normal, healthy skin is designed to look after itself by producing its own natural oils known as **NMFs** (Natural Moisturizing Factors). These will be maintained at a constant level in normal circumstances, and naturally increase in response to factors such as unaccustomed sun exposure, dryness or dehydration. However if you constantly slather your skin with layers of artificial moisturiser then your body's NMFs will assume that everything is ok and will sit back and enjoy the ride! They will become lazy. Over a period of time your skin will forget how to moisturize itself and will become very dry. And what do you (most likely) do in response? You slather on more moisturiser! Yet another vicious circle of events brought about by our interference with Mother Nature.

Before making the commitment to an holistic method of skincare, I had spent years applying lashings of moisturiser to my body every morning after showering and I remember that on the few occasions I let things slip, it took only five or six days for the skin on my legs (always the first to under-perform!) to become dry, flaky and patchy. I couldn't wait to get to work with the old exfoliating gloves (far too harsh, as I now realize) followed by lashings of lovely, rich, scented moisturiser that instantly put everything to rights again - not understanding that by doing this I was further compromising my skin's ability to repair and moisturize itself.

I also recall that my grandmother never used any kind of moisturiser on her face, always washing it in natural rainwater which she collected in a bucket! To the day she died she had beautiful, soft skin and a lovely complexion, which, as I have come across similar stories from other people, lends further credence to this theory.

There is however, another school of thought suggesting that our skin nowadays needs extra support due both to the massive increase in pollution from the environment around us, and to the toxic price it has to pay for our 21st century lifestyles. In theory I can agree absolutely with this argument. Yes, I think it very reasonable to believe that extra support might indeed be needed for today's "modern skin" but what if this support structure was to come from within, rather than from what is applied on the surface?

Unfortunately many people nowadays have been conditioned from quite an early age to use a moisturiser both on their face and on their body. The mere act of carrying out this daily routine provides them with a reassurance, a psychological dependence even, with the result that their skin is already compromised and has pretty much "retired from its duties", often before they reach middle age. This issue is compounded by the fact that many of the ingredients used in (usually but not always) cheaper skincare products, can actually make worse the very problem they are being used for in the first place.

For example, as is often the case, the molecules contained in **petroleum** and **mineral oil** (a derivative) are too large to permeate the skin's outer layers and so cannot be absorbed. They therefore sit rather greasily on the surface as a protective film which traps oil, toxins and waste products inside, contributing to breakouts in the skin and a general worsening of any existing skin conditions.

Glycerin, much loved by past generations for the lovely soft (albeit temporary) feel it gives to the skin, and still a basic ingredient in many of today's skincare products, is a humectant which means that unless there is a high humidity in the atmosphere of around 65% or above, it causes the skin to draw moisture from the basal layer of the epidermis to the surface at an unnatural rate, causing the keratinocytes there to dry up and therefore severely compromising cell renewal.

AHAs (alpha hydroxy acids) which caused a huge buzz in the beauty industry when they made their debut many years ago as anti-ageing products, promising the renewed, radiant and wrinkle-free skin of our youth, did in fact make a wonderful job of exfoliating away all the dead "rough stuff" from the skin's surface. Unfortunately however, they also did a wonderful job of removing the skin's own protective barrier, which as we have seen, is so vital in protecting its inner layers from toxins, free radicals and the like. AHAs are still around on the shelves at the moment.

Then of course there are all the synthetic chemicals and preservatives that we have already talked about in depth, like **propylene glycol**, yet another substance frequently used in moisturisers that can also be found in industrial products such as brake fluid and anti-freeze, and that is known to cause liver abnormalities and kidney damage. Check-out the ingredients on the packaging of as many products as you can next time you're in Boots or any other chemist, and see just how many times this substance turns up.

And the list goes on ...

All in all, it would appear that most moisturisers do more potential harm than good and by continuing to use them as an "easy" substitute for poor diet and lifestyle we are unwittingly putting our skin at risk.

Yes, applying any kind of moisturiser will indeed smooth and condition the cells on the surface, giving the illusion of plumped-up and radiant skin. *Yes,* the sensation of deliciously rich cream on the skin gives a certain feeling of decadence, like biting into a gooey cake (or whatever your poison happens to be!). But mostly, that is all it is, a mere comfort food for the skin with little nutritional value and the potential to do more harm than good in the long run. You only have to stop using it for a week or two to notice how your skin

– at best - has gone back to how it was before, and at worst is even drier and with an increased risk of frictional damage and wrinkle development.

As I mentioned earlier, big skincare companies rely quite heavily on the general ignorance of most consumers with regard both to the structure and function of their skin and to the small print on the bottle, and they would prefer to keep it that way. Knowledge and understanding is indeed the key, and the first important step forward in committing to a whole new and exciting way of caring for your skin. I hope you will enjoy the journey as much as I have done.

Section Three – THE PLAN

Introduction

If you have reached this far then **"Well Done"**, and thank you for persevering! I hope you have found the first two sections not only interesting and thought provoking, but also an inspiration to take that leap of faith into a whole exciting new world of skincare, a whole new level of understanding about how your body functions. Because it has all been in preparation for this, the final section of the book that tells you exactly what you need to do to "*smash that clock*" and call time on ageing skin for good. It really *is* just a simple matter of making certain lifestyle changes, and substituting good practices for bad, good foods for bad foods.

I first need you to think back to Chapter 6 in Part One – "Wanted, for crimes against your skin". An improved diet, on its own, is only one side of the coin and although this will obviously have a hugely positive impact on the general appearance and condition of your skin, its effect is obviously going to be compromised if you are smoking 20 cigarettes or drinking half a bottle of wine a day, if you continue to expose your skin to harmful toxins, chemicals and synthetic oils that are contained in your beauty products, household items or in the food you eat, if you are losing a large amount of weight too quickly, do not exercise, or suffer from stress, lack of sleep, chronic pain or too much sun exposure.

Every single one of these issues, if it applies to you, needs to be addressed. You may have several, you may only have one or two.

So firstly **identify them** and **write them down**, then **divide them into two categories**, those having short-term goals that you can realize quite quickly and with a minimum of effort, and those where it will take a longer time to achieve the desired results. For example, smoking and alcohol consumption will probably fall into the latter category for many people, as it is obviously unrealistic to expect anyone to give up overnight (although if you can, great, so much the better!).

Remember that while I want you to be amazed at the change in your appearance after as little as 10 weeks, this is a long-term plan designed to have a permanent impact on your general health and on the appearance of your skin.

It really is a case of "*Softly, softly catches the monkey*"! Tiny steps are better than no steps at all, (you have already taken the first major step by reading this book) and once the initial period of adjustment is over, you will be so delighted by the visible response of your skin that, like watching the pounds fall away on a diet, you will have all the incentive you need to carry on.

Do not make the mistake of thinking too much about the outcome, or giving yourself too-specific time scales, this only creates more pressure on you not to fail.

If it works for you, then by all means write down what you hope to have achieved at the end of each day/week/month/year, at the end of which time you can review and evaluate your progress.

However if you are still struggling with certain issues after, for example, a ten week period, then don't be too hard on yourself or be tempted to give up. You are gradually starting to replace all the negative elements of your lifestyle with positive ones, a journey where even just one step forward is one step closer to where you want to be, and one step further than you were the day before. No matter how slow your progress, you are still way ahead of everyone else who isn't trying so hold onto that thought.

If you have a bad day then "so what?" It happens, move on!

Make just one change at a time until you are relaxed and comfortable with it, and then move onto the next. Keep repeating this process until every issue on your list has been addressed.

As I suggested before, when it comes to dealing with household cleaning products, sink and drain un-blockers, tins and plastics containing BPAs, and anything else in the home you wish to banish to the re-cycle bin, then work on a gradual replacement basis. Every time you run out of something, simply replace it with a more eco-friendly and less harmful alternative. This keeps any stress out of the exercise and will hopefully help in your resolve to make the home a safer place for you and your family.

I would suggest also, that you **continue to use a minimal amount of moisturiser** on your skin throughout this transitional period, but switch to a natural product free from fragrance and synthetic preservatives. Once your skin is responding well to your improved lifestyle, then you can think about leaving your moisturiser off altogether, or using the smallest amount of one containing ingredients that you know will support your skin from the inside. By now, however, this will not be a necessity but the icing on the cake, the final gilding of the lily, as it were!

So find below a list of all the main issues that are known to be seriously damaging to your skin in both the short and the long-term, together with some suggested ways in which to address them. Read, learn and prepare for action!

Part One: 15 deadly enemies of your skin revisited …

Top Tips to help you tackle them *once and for all*

Smoking

If you do only one thing after reading this book, and you a smoker then **please** let that one thing be that you give up smoking for good. Of all the ways that can not only slow down but also reverse the ageing process, giving up smoking is the one that will give you the most amazing and quickly visible results. The overall benefits to your health and to your skin will be inestimable.

1. List the **reasons** why you want/need to stop, and keep this list with you at all times to help you stay focused. Maybe have with it, a **picture or photo** of an ashtray piled high with unsavory looking cigarette ends, so that every time you look at it you are reminded of what you have deposited into your lungs and what it is doing to your health and to your skin.

2. Set **small goals** if this works for you, like getting through the first day, week or month. You may only be able to think about cutting down at first, and this is ok. Remember, every step - however small, is one step further forward than you were this time last week. Without meaning to sound patronizing, every time you are tempted and resist, give yourself a reward – maybe something special to eat or drink that you might not normally indulge in, or that latest CD you've been meaning to buy.

3. **Save** the money you would have spent on cigarettes, in a piggy bank (there is something addictive in the fact that you can't see inside so have absolutely no idea of exactly how much it is you're accumulating!). Decide beforehand what you will use it for (new clothes, perhaps, or maybe a break away) and this will be an added incentive to give up.

4. **Talk** to family and friends and make them aware of what you are doing – it is so much harder to back down once others know what you are intending to do, as you run a serious risk of ending up with egg on your face if you don't follow it through!

5. **Empty** your house, car, desk drawers, pockets etc of cigarettes, lighters and ashtrays. Fill them instead, with little packs of healthy snacks or sugar free gum.

6. If anyone else in your household smokes and is unwilling to join you in giving up, then you will have to come to some sort of mutual arrangement between you as to how you are going to compromise - although **it really does help to have the support of a partner or family member**. If that support is not forthcoming then resolve to be even stronger and more determined to prove that you can do this on your own.

7. Think of things you can **occupy** yourself with at times when you would normally be having a cigarette, or when you feel stressed. *Stress Balls* are a great way to instantly relieve stress and give your hands something to do. You can buy them on Amazon for under five pounds, all different colours and with funny/smiley faces etc! Also, to begin with, you will probably need to avoid any situation where you know you will be tempted to light up.

8. Consider **Nicotine Replacement Therapy** such as skin patches (which work via the method of trans-dermal absorption which we mentioned earlier), lozenges, chewing gum, or mouth and nasal sprays, all of which can be purchased over the counter or obtained on prescription. They can help your body deal with any withdrawal symptoms by providing it with what is essentially a "fix" of nicotine.

9. Try the **E-Cigarette**. This may particularly help those who see smoking as a part of their identity, part of who they are, and as such find it really difficult to summon up the courage to stop.

I gave up smoking some years ago before e-cigs were on the market (one of those annoying individuals who literally decided on a date to give up and stopped practically overnight) but having tried e-cigarettes purely out of curiosity I would recommend anyone to give them a go. They look really cool, give you something to do with your hands at a time when you might be in danger of losing your resolve, and have a familiarity about them that is comforting. Plus, at the time of writing, they can be smoked in most public places. The only reservations I have are that:

○ Most E-cigs contain the chemical **propylene glycol** in the vapour, and while it may only be a very small amount, as we have seen it is the gradual build-up in your body as a result of prolonged exposure to toxic chemicals that causes the damage. However e-cigs have none of the 4000 or so other toxins and cancer-causing chemicals contained in regular cigarettes, so are still by far the healthier option.

○ If you are in the habit of inhaling deeply, then it is possible you may inhale some of the liquid nicotine with its associated side-effects; however e-cigs contain none of the tobacco and tar that is in regular cigarettes.

○ The repetitious pursing of the lips can lead, as with any cigarettes, to the development of fine lines above the upper lip. However, the overall advantages of not smoking will far outweigh the few disadvantages of e-cigarettes if this is the only way that works for you to give up.

10. If you have tried all of the above and are still having difficulty in giving up, then there are medicines available that can double your chance of success – especially when combined with a Support Service like **NHS Smoke-Free**, or **Quit**. The numbers of your local branches can be obtained from your GP or from any Stop Smoking helpline, and they will provide you with expert advice, ongoing support and practical guidance.

The two most widely used medications, *Bupropion* (*Zyban*) and *Varenicline* (*Champix*), are available on prescription as a two to three month course that decreases both the urge to smoke and any withdrawal symptoms. However you need to think carefully about whether this is the right solution for you, as they do come with side effects one of the most common of which is depression. Your local support service will talk to you and advise you on this.

11. The use of **Visualization Techniques** may help you to resist temptation. Picture the network of blood vessels within your system, freed from all its accumulated gunge and

with your blood now able to flow unimpeded to all parts of your body, carrying its supply of essential nutrients, vitamins and minerals to your vital organs and to your skin. *Picture* how luminous and radiant your skin will be, and how much younger and more vibrant you will both look and feel. Research has shown that those who are able to vividly imagine the result they are aiming for, are those ones least likely to give up on their quest.

12. Finally, you need to be able to deal with any **mental or physical stress** caused through your body's adjustment to decreased nicotine levels. You will find tips and advice for this later in this chapter under "Stress".

Alcohol

When it comes to alcohol, cutting down does **not** necessarily mean giving up for those who enjoy a drink (unless of course, you have a serious problem with alcohol).

If you *are* able to give up completely then the difference in your skin will be immeasurable - and indeed it may be really beneficial to abstain for a period of time just so you know you *can*. This exercise can be quite empowering as it puts you in complete control at the same time as knowing it need not be forever.

However even to cut down will still give you visible results, especially when in combination with the other elements of an internal and holistic approach to health and beauty - and in fact it has been proven that one or two small glasses of red wine with a meal can help protect your blood vessels and your heart due to the anti-oxidant *reservatrol* that it contains.

Try any or all of the suggestions below to help you to better control your alcohol consumption while still being able to enjoy a drink. Your current drinking habits should obviously be the guiding factor in how far you want to play this.

1. Write down the **reasons** why you want to give up or cut down on alcohol, and keep the list with you at all times.

2. Decide what your **expectations** are going to be, for example might it work better for you to aim for a couple less drinks a day (depending on your average daily consumption), or to have two or three days a week when you give your body a complete break from alcohol and then resume just a modest amount. If, as with myself, you find that you do actually feel better after a break, this may well be an incentive to give up or to even more drastically cut down at some point in the future.

3. It may help to **keep an informal diary** of what you drink in a week as you can use this

as a baseline against which to measure your progress.

4.   Identify the **situations** where you are most likely to want/need a drink, and the friends with whom you are most likely to have a drink, then plan ahead as to how you will keep to your resolve but still have a good time.

5.   As with the issue of smoking, **talk** to your family and friends and ask them to respect your decisions and not to try to talk you out of them. People can be funny, sometimes, in the way they don't like it when one of "the gang" suddenly tries to break out of the mold and do something different, but at the end of the day they will respect you more for sticking to your guns rather than giving in at the first cries of, "Oh go on, have another, it won't hurt you!" etc. You just have to learn how to say "No" politely but firmly, and trust me, you'll be the one to have the last laugh!

6.   You need to stay **hydrated** when you drink, and this is really important. Alcohol is a well-known cause of dehydration which, quite apart from anything else, has drastic and unattractive effects upon your skin.

     Make it a habit, therefore, to drink a large glass of water beforehand so that you don't use your alcoholic drink to quench your thirst, and then have regular drinks of water throughout the evening. Any restaurant or pub will give you a glass of tap-water (usually free), or if you prefer you could sip your way through a couple of glasses of sparkling water. Dress it up with ice if you like, and a slice or two of lime or lemon to add some "zing"!

At home I like to drink water with a good squeeze of fresh lime juice, and find this really refreshing. It also clears your palate in a similar way to sorbet in between the courses of a rich meal, which means that you are less likely to want to smoke/drink/eat fatty foods.

I'm very aware that experts are now telling us not to drink a lot of citrus juice because it softens tooth enamel, but if it helps you drink less alcohol then I think this weighs in its favour, plus it's a good source of Vitamin C. Just try to avoid cleaning your teeth for half an hour to an hour afterwards, to give the enamel a chance to harden again.

7.   It is always a good idea to **dilute** your drinks with your favourite mixer. I'm a wine drinker, and genuinely enjoy mixing white or red wine with tonic water to make a refreshing spritzer. It not only makes your drink last longer but means that the alcohol content is absorbed more quickly (so you are less likely

to have an unpleasant hangover!). Opt for the low-calorie versions as regular mixers contain extra sugar! Still water is even better.as containing no artificial sweetener.

8. If you don't like to dilute your drinks then try alternating a soft drink with each alcoholic one. Avoid fizzy carbonated drinks such as coke however, as these too are full of added sugar and have no health benefits whatsoever.

9. Get into the habit of **drinking slowly**, replacing your glass after a few sips rather than keeping it in your hand. Try to focus on conversation and/or any other activities that may be going on rather than on your drink, and drink at your own pace, not everyone else's. To be firm over this is a sign of strength of character, and whatever they may say, deep down your friends will respect you for it.

10. At home remember "**Out of sight is out of mind**", so try not to leave temptation lying around and only buy drink as you need it. This is obviously difficult if you and your partner/spouse entertain a lot, as the drinks cabinet will no doubt be kept permanently well-stocked, but limiting your purchase works well for some people.

You could start by buying just a bottle of wine rather than a box (I find a box of wine is a false economy anyway as, like a box of chocolates, if it's there I keep chipping away until there's no more left!). I often just buy a miniature bottle of wine in the evening, which effectively limits my intake to the 187mls or so that are in the bottle.

11. Try buying drinks with a **lower alcoholic content**, as this will equate to actively and dramatically reducing your daily/weekly intake.

12. **Use smaller glasses**. Research has shown that those using wider or deeper wine glasses pour themselves more wine than those pouring into a smaller glass, especially if that glass is in the hand rather than placed on the table. I have a collection of attractive green-stemmed Germanic glasses, all acquired from local charity shops, which hold around 125mls of wine and have always been a talking point with friends.

13. And finally, if you drink for relaxation then try to find **alternative ways of relaxing** on some occasions, for instance a lovely long, scented bath with candles and your favourite music (old hat I know, but it works!), a good book, a new hobby or, at the rather more bizarre end of the scale the thing that invariably works for me as a total distraction

is to start sorting out old photos or papers, bills etc. that need to be thrown away. Once started I find this utterly absorbing and therapeutic as only the act of de-cluttering can be! I also make sure that I have some really delicious non-alcoholic drinks in the fridge to provide the "treat" factor, as often the simple act of pouring (any kind of) drink is all that is needed to satisfy your mind that your body is relaxing.

Fatty Foods

As you will now realize from earlier chapters, your body (and most definitely your skin) needs a certain amount of fat, including some saturated fat, in order to function. Apart from providing a source of energy, it protects, insulates and facilitates the transportation and absorption of important vitamins around your body. It also provides essential fatty acids that your body is unable to manufacture for itself.

However most of us eat far more than we should of the **wrong** type of fat which, apart from being a serious health risk, at about nine calories for every gram of fat is a major factor in weight gain and obesity.

On the face of it, the most straightforward way to reduce your fat intake is to substitute low-fat foods for high-fat ones and this is the advice most often given, particularly with regard to weight loss. However if you remember, I spoke at length earlier about the dangers of low-fat diets, and how they are a killer for your health - and especially your skin - with few, if any, health benefits. Dull, lank hair and dry, rough or scaly skin are some of the signs of a diet deficient in beneficial fats.

I have listed below some ways that I personally would recommend, to help eliminate an excess of bad fats from your diet, while including enough of the good fats to promote a nourished and beautiful skin.

1. Rather than using low-fat spreads include moderate amounts of **butter** in your diet, spreading thinly on bread, toast or crackers and using plenty of healthy filling/topping. This is actually much better for you, as being a wholesome and natural food butter does a far better job than its low fat and cholesterol-lowering counterparts in suppressing hunger pangs and reducing the appetite.

   Butter is also an excellent source of vitamin A, whereas research has shown that the supposedly healthier low-fat alternatives can actually inhibit the absorption of certain vitamins owing to the amount of plant sterols that they contain (these are part of the natural cell structures in plants and have a similar composition to our human cholesterol). I always use *organic butter* as I believe this to be a far healthier alternative to non-organic.

2. **Full-fat milk** has also received bad press due to our perception of it as being a high-fat food item. However with between just 3.7% and 5% fat in every 100ml, unless you regularly consume vast quantities it will not make a significant difference to your daily fat intake and is more nutritious than skimmed or semi-skimmed milks which contain respectively around 0.1% and 1.5% of fat per 100ml.

It is rich in the nutrients and vitamins that your skin loves, particularly the fat-soluble vitamins A, D, E and K that are found in the cream and which, amongst other things, are front players in the war against free radicals.

It is a leading source of the healthy polyunsaturated fatty acids that are so good for your heart, especially *organic milk* where the levels of these fatty acids have been found to be significantly and consistently higher. This is reportedly due to the fact that "organic" cows are allowed full access to pasture and therefore eat a natural diet rather than processed corn and grains favoured by non-organic farmers.

Milk is also rich in amino acids which help keep the skin's cells plumped up with moisture, and its anti-oxidant properties help fight free radicals and improve collagen production, and therefore elasticity, in the skin.

What I'm saying here is that, if you prefer full-fat milk, then it's okay to drink it in moderation as its powerhouse of vitamins are good for your general health and nourishing for your skin.

It does contain 4.7% natural sugars in the form of lactose, which, although processed in a slightly different way in your body to sucrose and fructose, could potentially raise insulin levels if drunk in excessive amounts.

If, therefore, you drink an awful lot of milk in a day (by which I mean more than just in tea and coffee and on your breakfast cereal) or if you are lactose intolerant, you should consider including *coconut* or *unsweetened almond milk* as a portion of your overall intake. Both are delicious on cereal and make lovely porridge. But don't avoid full fat milk altogether because you think it is bad for you. Like most things, in sensible amounts it is not and your skin will love it!

I have deliberately not included soy milk here as an alternative because, although a good source of healthy Omega 3 essential fatty acids and protein, as I mentioned earlier it contains both natural and added toxins, including cane sugar as a replacement for lactose, so is not as healthy as was previously thought. Additionally it contains only around a quarter of the amount of calcium as that found in cow's milk. However due to the positive health benefits it *does* offer, if you like soy milk and want to drink it, then just bear in mind its downsides and limit your intake to a minimum.

3. **Avoid fatty cuts of meat**. Trim off any visible fat and remove all skin before cooking.

4. Whenever you can, **opt for white meats such as chicken and turkey** which are lower in saturated fat than red meats like lamb or beef. You should look for locally produced/organic/outdoor reared produce as this is the only way to avoid the added water, salt and chemicals now pumped into most of the meat that we are being sold. **Seafood** is also a good option, especially grilled or baked fish.

5. **Grill, bake (... or even better) poach or steam** food rather than frying, so that you won't be adding any extra fat. This does not apply to stir fries which are both nutritious and healthy. If you do fry, use a small quantity of good quality, unrefined olive oil. Not only is this healthy but it requires a smaller amount in the cooking process (you will use less by pouring a measured amount from a tablespoon rather than by tipping it straight out of the bottle).

6. **Make sure that you only ever cook the oil over a very moderate heat and *never allow***

it to burn. By doing this you will lose much of the nutritional content and also risk changing the structure of the oil, a process that creates free radicals which can damage not only your body's cells but the DNA they contain. Add a splash of water or wine to the pan during cooking, both to reduce the heat and, in the case of wine, add a little extra flavour.

If you prefer, you could substitute extra virgin coconut oil (available from health stores) which gives a lovely flavour when used in the cooking of pancakes, stir fries etc. It makes your kitchen smell lovely too! Coconut oil is a very stable and healthy cooking oil with anti-oxidant, anti-inflammatory and anti-viral properties – *and it will not change structure over a high heat*. I highly recommend it.

7. When you make stews, casseroles or curries with red meat, try using just a little **less meat** and adding bulk in the form of extra vegetables. Always skim any surplus fat off the top before serving.

8. If you eat a lot of hard cheese, try switching to one that has a **lower fat content** such as Gouda or Edam, or alternating these with lesser amounts of your favourite extra-mature Cheddar. Acquire the habit of **slicing your cheese thinly** rather than cutting off large chunks, or use a small amount of **grated cheese** in a salad or as a filling.

As before, we are not talking here about a lifetime of deprivation but more about making smart choices and compromises to your lifestyle that are sustainable in the long term.

"Whole" foods that contain saturated fat such as butter and cheese, are far better for you (especially when derived from grass-fed animals rather than those fed on corn or soy products) than processed low-fat foods containing a bucket-load of sugar. In fact this fat content can be very beneficial for your skin. You just need to learn to go easy on the amount you eat so as not to risk causing health issues such as weight gain, which will actually compromise your skin's integrity. Once again it comes down to *Balance, Balance, Balance*.

9. When eating out avoid meals that you know are loaded with **hidden fats** such as baltis and kormas (Indian cuisine), sweet and sour (Chinese), or creamy pastas and risottos (Italian).

   ○ Opt for **tomato-based dishes** when you can, and choose whole-grain (if available) or plain steamed rice, rather than fried.

   ○ Even though most rice contains a whopping eight to nine spoonfuls of sugar in one heaped bowl (eight to nine spoonfuls that will end up being stored as fat in your body), steamed rice is a reluctantly better option than fried as at least you are not consuming all the additional fat used in the cooking, alongside. Worth remembering too, that basmati rice is a low AGE carbohydrate ...

o **However,** as with white bread, white rice has been stripped of almost all its vitamins, minerals, fibre and nutrients, **which makes it hard for your body to digest and process** – so if there is no alternative then try having a smaller serving.

o *Brown rice, in its more natural and unrefined form, is a far better option* and you should opt for this if there is a choice available. I find brown rice to be so much tastier, although once it's covered in sauce I can't see that you would notice much difference anyway!

10. **Don't smother your salads with creamy dressings**. Instead experiment with making your own to taste, using simple ingredients like extra-virgin olive oil, fresh lemon and vinegar as a base or simply add a squeeze of lime/lemon juice with some freshly ground black pepper, or a drizzle of reduced-sugar balsamic vinegar. Not only is this healthier and better for your skin, but it allows you to enjoy the separate tastes and the crunch factor of all those lovely salad ingredients.

If you really prefer a ready-made dressing then you need to get out there and compare what's on offer in your local shops and supermarkets. There are healthy alternatives if you look for them: for instance some supermarkets stock the *"Naturally Righteous"* range of salad dressings, all of which are made from 100% natural ingredients with no added flavours, colours or preservatives, and are GM free.

Their "*ginger and toasted sesame*" dressing is Japanese inspired, and has minimal levels of fat, salt and sugar, as does the "*lemon and mustard*". Alternatively they offer an oil-free "*caper and peppercorn*" dressing which is fat-free, gluten-free and soy-free and yet contains a minimum of sugar and salt. All are totally delicious.

11. **Avoid processed and packaged meals and pre-packed sandwiches** which almost always contain large amounts of fat and sugar, not to mention additives, preservatives, and processed salt. Not only this but much of the nutritional content of "ready" meals is lost through heavy pre-cooking followed by re-heating again in the microwave or oven at home.

If you do have occasion to buy them then look at local farm shops and garden centres which sometimes stock locally produced packaged meals. They may contain lower fat/sugar levels than the majority of those from the supermarket, and if they happen to be organically produced then they'll most certainly be healthier. Search online also, for specialist companies producing organic meals, such as "*Planet Organic*". It is nevertheless important to realize that *just because a product is organic does not automatically guarantee that it will have low fat and sugar levels*. Quorn and vegetable based meals are generally better than those which contain meat. **However ...**

12. **... ALWAYS read the nutrition labels** which will tell you the amount of fat and saturated fat that is present in each 100gms. As a guide, the total fat content is *high* if more than 17.5g of fat per 100g, and *low* if 3g or below. The saturated fat content is *high* if more than 5g per 100g and *low* if 1.5g or below.

If colour coding is used then RED = High, AMBER = Medium and GREEN = Low. My advice is to write this down on a little card (do the same also, for sugar and salt) and keep it in your purse at all times. You are then able to quickly and easily check what's in any product (save for the unpackaged ones) that you buy.

13. Above all, apart from the occasional treat, for instance when out with friends, **avoid, or drastically cut down your consumption of**

those foods that you know are laden with hidden and deadly trans-fats. These include takeaways (especially curries and all fried foods), bought cakes, biscuits, cookies and pies, all processed meats, sausage rolls, fried breakfasts etc. These all spell eventual suicide, both for your health and for your skin.

Instead **develop a taste for the good fats** in foods like *avocados* (deliciously creamy!), *nuts and seeds* (make great snacks!) and *oily fish* (tasty and versatile), gradually substituting these lovely foods each time you are tempted to indulge in an unhealthy alternative.

14. You can still enjoy a cooked breakfast at home occasionally, but *grill* your food rather than frying it, and trim as much excess fat as you can off your bacon beforehand. If you have breakfast out, ask if your food can be grilled instead of fried. Grilling, along with frying, can result in the production of AGEs (as mentioned in Section 1 Chapter 6). However it is still by far the better option so long as you grill your food lightly – it's the charred, brown bits that result from overcooking that cause the problems.

15. Make your own curries at home using healthy, organic and unprocessed ingredients and invite friends round to share them. Let your curry evenings become legend!

16. Bake your own cakes substituting unprocessed and healthier ingredients for *unhealthy* ones. Once your eating habits have been reformed and you can see the wonderful changes visible in your skin, you may well decide that actually no, you really don't have the taste for these sweeter "comfort-type" foods anymore.

17. The general message therefore, is that you need to re-educate your taste buds and learn how to make informed and healthy choices that will have long-term benefits for your general well-being and for your skin. Focus upon the good fats, maintain a moderate consumption of saturated fats, and banish as many trans fats from your diet as you can.

Sugar

As discussed at length in an earlier chapter of this book, sugar is an independent and highly significant risk factor to your general health, now considered to be on a par with cigarette smoke and excessive alcohol consumption. In dietary terms it is a far greater enemy of your skin than are (previously accused) saturated fats.

Since waging war on saturated fats for more than three decades, the food industry has responded by adding extra sugar to low fat products to compensate for the resulting lack of taste, and apart from its staggeringly damaging effects on every bodily system, it is very, very addictive.

Here are my top tips on how to train your taste buds to become accustomed to a great deal less sugar in your diet, with a view to ultimately eliminating the vast majority of those foods that contain it.

1. **Avoid all low-fat foods** which are generally loaded with sugar. This is considered necessary on the part of the manufacturers, as it makes the foods taste good in the absence of fat.

   Weight loss diets, while primarily helping you to lose weight, are also often good for your general health and vitality as they usually include a high proportion of fruits and vegetables and recommend that you drink plenty of water. However on the down-side is the issue of low fat foods which the majority of diet plans recommend that you eat. These are no good for you, they are loaded with sugar.

   If you follow the plan that I set out at the end - although it is not primarily aimed at weight loss - over time you will find that you are losing weight without even trying, as your system unclogs and becomes free of its build-up of toxins and all the "bad" fats and sugars that contribute to an un-healthy body and a dull, lack-lustre skin. Food for thought …

2. **Read**, read, read the labels. Sugar comes in many guises, the most common ones of which

end in "ose", for example sucrose, dextrose, fructose, maltose and glucose. Other common ingredients which should set the alarm bells ringing are corn syrup, honey (although this does contain some valuable nutrients and enzymes to compensate), hydrolysed starch, invert sugar, and fruit juice concentrate.

You need to look for "Carbohydrates (of which sugars...)" on the nutrition label. A high sugar content is 22.5g or above per 100g, and a low one is 5g or less per 100g. Obviously a medium sugar content falls in between the two. If colour coding is used, then as with fat content, RED = High, AMBER = Medium and GREEN = Low.

3. **Cut down on your consumption of alcohol**, some of which has a surprisingly high sugar content. Red wine, dry sherry and champagne contain only a minimal amount in comparison with white wine, cider and sweet sherry. Gin, whisky and vodka also contain only small traces of sugar, but the danger is in the mixers you put with them - while a pint of real ale contains up to nine spoonfuls of sweet stuff.

4. **Avoid the majority of "ready meals"**, both sweet and savoury. Although the sugar content will vary from brand to brand, most will be quite high.

I was checking out a raspberry and coconut sponge pudding recently, from a leading supermarket – sounded very healthy, you know, raspberry, coconut, both delicious, healthy- sounding ingredients - oh, and no added flavour or colourings, an added incentive. However on reading the label I found that it had 12.4g of fat per 25g serving, and **a massive 35.8g of sugar**, plus an assortment of raising agents, flour acidity regulators and a gelling agent to boot. As I said above, **do read the labels**.

5. Check out your local farm shops and garden centres - some of which may offer a range of locally prepared meals that have a lower fat/sugar content than those on sale elsewhere. However *there is no substitute for preparing your own delicious meals with "whole", and known ingredients* at home. Mediterranean peoples do this all the time and are conspicuously healthy and with lovely clear skin.

Note: if you are looking for inspiration to start growing your own vegetables/fruit, or to create your own meals from the freshest ingredients, then you could do worse than read those of Elizabeth Adler's books that are set in the South of France such as "The Hotel Riviera", "Invitation to Provence" and "There's Something About St.Tropez". Trust me, by the time you've got to the end you'll be an absolute convert (apart from the fact that they're all damn good mystery stories with interesting and "fun" characters!). The food, and the preparation of it, is described in such a way as to almost make it an art form!

6. **Beware of breakfast cereals**. However healthy they pretend to be most of them are heavily laden with sugar. "Special K" is a prime example of a low-fat "healthy" option that, at around six spoonfuls of sugar in every average bowl, is quite patently not healthy at all. You may be surprised to hear that muesli is equally as bad if not worse.

   Opt for whole-grain varieties as opposed to anything honey-coated, frosted or containing clusters, berries or (God save us) chocolate. Alternatively switch to porridge (currently bang on trend) which is a deliciously nutritious way to start the day and as a substitute ticks all the boxes.

7. Top with **fresh fruit** rather than refined sugar, as this will satisfy your need for something sweet, or add a drizzle of *treacle* (yes, really!) which, as a mere by-product of the process that produces refined sugar, is actually extremely rich in minerals and B vitamins to offset its sugar content.

   o *Blackstrap molasses*, an un-crystallized dark syrupy residue from the back-end of the refining process, is a great source of vitamins, minerals and iron, and gives a sumptuous dark hue and a delicious caramel flavour when used in home-made cake and pudding mixes or to sweeten porridge, as does *malt extract*.

○ *Maple syrup* too, is a surprisingly rich source of essential nutrients such as manganese and zinc, plus over 30 recently discovered compounds that are beneficial to your health and that make it a more viable option – in small amounts - than refined sugar.

8. **Avoid coca cola and all sports drinks** – you might as well be drinking liquidized sugar, as a standard can of coke contains around eight to nine spoonfuls of the stuff! Some high energy drinks such as Red Bull have also been reported to contain large doses of caffeine, plus added chemicals that are normally only present in your body in minute concentrations.

9. **Limit your consumption of sauces**, ketchups and dressings, low fat mayonnaise, baked beans, mushy peas and many bought soups, most of which contain hidden sugar. Scour your supermarket shelves or small local shops for smaller "niche" brands that have a reduced level of sugar, and that are made from natural ingredients.

Even big brand-name companies are becoming increasingly aware of the needs of their more health-conscious customers, and we are slowly beginning to see an attempt being made by them, to meet these needs.

o **HP**, for example, offers a reduced salt/reduced sugar brown sauce with no added colours, flavourings or preservatives.

o The **French's** brand also, has some similarly healthier options including a classic yellow mustard, while **Kikkoman's** soy sauce is naturally brewed and contains only four ingredients: soybeans, wheat, salt and water. It has no artificial colours or flavourings, and a low sugar content of 3.9gm per 100ml.

o The **Sanchi** range has little if any sugar in any of its products, but is not always as readily available on the shelves as is Kikkoman.

10. **Always, but Always** check the content of all three main offenders, namely sugar, fat and salt, as any product that is low in one may well be very high in another. **Heinz**, for instance, has an organic tomato ketchup on the shelves which, although undeniably a healthier option than its regular bog-standard ketchup, still

contains a whopping 4.6gm of sugar per 15ml serving.

If you are unable to find a satisfactory alternative, then when it comes to most soups, sauces, salad dressings (including mayonnaise) and stocks it is worth taking that little extra time to make your own, especially where you can make a large amount and freeze for another time.

Note: Any mass-produced products with "sweet and sour", "sweet chilli", "balsamic" or "caramelized" in the title, will be high in sugars, so avoid these tantalizingly described but rather less than healthy options.

11. **Cut down** the amount of cordials and fruit juices you drink. Many juice drinks contain extra sugar, and even the "no added sugar" varieties are high in fructose. Opt in moderation (as excessive amounts can wear away the enamel on your teeth) for natural fruit juices that are additive-free and *not* made from concentrate which is high in natural fruit sugars.

12. To protect your teeth yet further, try **diluting** your juice with some water. Better still eat fresh fruit which, despite its inherent natural sugar content, also contains a full complement of vitamins, minerals and essential fibre and so

offers more health benefits than just the juice on its own.

If you use tinned fruit then obviously opt for fruit "in natural juice" rather than in syrup, but fresh fruit is always by far the better choice to make.

Note: although I normally try to eat fruit on an empty stomach to aid its digestion, it is worth remembering that an apple after a meal will naturally help to neutralize dental plaque acids, as will carrot or celery, or a small piece of cheese.

13. Try to **cut down or eliminate completely**, all shop-bought biscuits, cakes, pastries and pies etc, which are full of highly processed ingredients. If you have a very sweet tooth and find it hard to cut these from your diet, then do your own baking at home where you can control the type and amount of fat, sugar and salt that you use.

14. Baking is a lovely skill to have and, thanks to all the cookery programs and competitions on TV, has been re-invented as a really current and cool thing to be able to do. Most cakes and puddings however, apart from any ingredients you might add such as dried fruit, nuts, or grated carrot or parsnip to impart natural sweetness, will still have relatively little nutritional value as far as your health and your

skin are concerned, so do eat very much in moderation or as an occasional treat for you and the family.

15. An alternative to processed sugar for use in making cakes, puddings, marinades and chutneys, is **Billington's Molasses**, a natural, unrefined cane sugar available in most of the larger supermarkets. **Golden granulated** is available in the same range. Waitrose also sell their own brand of **unrefined soft and muscavado sugars.** Although significantly better to use than their highly processed counterparts, these products are, of course, still sugar, but if you find it difficult initially to adjust to substituting natural sweeteners (of which more below) then it is a better option than to continue to use regular, refined sugar containing just empty calories.

16. You could also try **halving the amount of sugar you would normally use,** and this should work very well with most recipes.

17. However always be on the lookout for healthier alternatives … browse your local health food stores and delicatessens to see what's on offer. Once you acquire this habit, it will become totally addictive!

18. You may find it helpful to decide on a plan for eating desserts and puddings. Maybe only have one at weekends when it will become

more of a treat - and if you are eating out then avoid pastry, crumble, steamed puds or fancy ice-cream based concoctions, opting instead for a lighter dessert or some cheese and fruit. At home do not keep ice-cream or other desserts in the fridge unless you have a cast-iron willpower!

19. Consider **replacing refined sugars** used in baking and hot drinks with **Stevia** (which comes directly from the Stevia plant native to Paraguay, and has been used as a sweetener for at least 40 years in Japan and South America). It is to be found in local health food stores, larger supermarkets and online.

   ○ I mostly use Stevia sweetener from Holland & Barrett (I also recently found some less than half price in Home Bargains!) and find it to be great in hot drinks, particularly the small "sugar" lumps (if you can get them) or the little sticks or sachets. You will need to experiment with the amounts you use as Stevia is much sweeter than sugar, but once you get it right then this is a very easy change to make.

   ○ An added bonus with Stevia is that it doesn't raise your blood sugar (brilliant news for diabetics) and is completely natural, unlike most other branded products that contain artificial sweeteners such as aspartame and sucralose - both of which have strong links to neurological and gastro-intestinal damage, and endocrine imbalance. And yes, I have read adverse reports on this product also, but if you have a sweet tooth and can't give up sugar, then I believe it to be a better option than either refined sugar or your regular sweeteners.

○ The brand I use from Holland & Barrett contains only Stevia extract, inulin and an anti-caking agent, with NO artificial colours or flavours, NO preservative, NO starch, NO corn, NO milk, NO lactose, NO soya, NO gluten, NO wheat, NO yeast, No fish and NO porcine. Equally you could try **Truvia**, manufactured by Silver Spoon – this also comes in handy sachets equivalent to a teaspoon of sugar, and I can honestly not taste the difference in hot drinks.

20. For baking I slightly prefer **"Total Sweet"** (Healthy Nature Ltd), available from health shops. The sole ingredient in this is *Xylitol*, naturally found in fruits and vegetables, and although at the end of the day it is still a form of sugar, it contains 75% less available carbohydrate, is suitable for diabetics and is aspartame-free. It can be used more or less spoonful for spoonful like regular sugar, and does not have the slightly bitter aftertaste that you sometimes get with stevia products.

21. And finally, I also sometimes use premium **agave nectar** (light and mild) from The Groovy Food Company, a product which is available on the shelves in some of the larger supermarkets (try Waitrose).

   o Agave nectar is derived from the succulent-type Agave plant. It looks like runny honey, and I have used it very successfully in baking, to add a little extra sweetness to cooked fruit, and as a substitute for regular honey when drizzled over Greek yoghurt.

   o **Note:** agave nectar contains quite a high proportion of fructose which, in excessive amounts, is thought to increase the amount of fatty acids circulating in the blood. However you would need to consume an awful lot of it for this to happen, and as long as you use only modest amounts you should have no problems. It is still a good alternative for diabetics as it does not raise insulin levels in the body.

22. As I've said before, **it's all about making healthier choices.** If, for example, you want to make a fruit crumble, try sweetening the fruit with just a little agave nectar and make only a thin layer of crumble from a mix of spelt, buckwheat or other unprocessed flour and oats, with some butter. Serve with single cream or a dollop of Greek yoghurt rather than custard.

23. **Keep most chocolate as an occasional treat**. Dark chocolate with a high percentage of cocoa solids (70-75% cacao) is a far healthier choice than milk or white chocolate, both of which have a whole spoonful of sugar lurking in each tiny square! It contains unique anti-oxidants called *flavanols* which reduce inflammation, naturally hydrate your skin and provide a low level of protection against the sun's UV rays. It is also a source of *Zinc.*

For these reasons dark chocolate is actually good for you in modest amounts, for example a couple of squares after a meal in place of a pudding. *Add a glass of red wine with its reservatrol content, for a potent nightly cocktail of anti-oxidants!*

Do not, however, keep bars of chocolate around the house where you can easily find them (the freezer is a good place, as frozen chocolate lasts so much longer) and have only one or two squares rather than the whole bar.

24. **Make your own smoothies** with a small amount of your choice of fresh fruit blended with plain, full fat yoghurt, and keep a jug in the fridge for when you need something sweet and to help prevent cravings.

Although there are of course, *natural* sugars in the fruit, it is still a far better and healthier replacement for soft or fizzy drinks with all their *added* sugars and chemical preservatives and I think it unrealistic to cut it from your diet altogether. Or have little snacks like fresh fruit, nuts or seeds (I love sunflower seeds and can eat them by the handful) to munch on in a crisis!

25. **Keep your blood sugar levels stable** and **reduce your cravings** even further by eating plenty of protein (for example *white meat, fish, tofu, eggs, full-fat yoghurt or beans and pulses*), good fats (*avocados, nuts and seeds*) and lots of lovely *vegetables*.

26. **Cinnamon** is also considered a good remedy, and is easily added to your diet by sprinkling over stewed fruit or mixing with yoghurt or smoothies. Taking cinnamon before a meal can reportedly control your blood sugars quite dramatically from that meal, as can drinking a little lemon juice.

27. As you cut down more and more on sugary, starchy foods, your body will start to adapt to your new and improved diet, resulting in a feeling of vitality and well-being, and a radiant, relaxed skin. The ultimate goal is of course, to eliminate sugar from your diet altogether, or to cut it down to a bare minimum. *If you do even just this one thing, then you will both see and feel a dramatic difference.*

28. Although fresh fruit contains natural sugar (and yes, I agree, sugar is sugar whatever the source), remember that it is still a far healthier choice than foods containing the same amount of *added* sugars due to the wealth of nutrients it contains.

29. There is a school of thought currently that recommends cutting every last atom of sugar from your diet, including, in some cases, **all** fresh or dried fruit. While I respect this viewpoint and do not in any way dispute its benefits, my own opinion is that fruits offer such a wealth and such a broad spectrum of nutrients, are such a wonderfully rich source of essential dietary fibre and are so versatile and delicious, that to cut them out of your diet would be a tragedy. *For most people this would also be unsustainable in the long-term.*

30. **The sugars you should absolutely be looking to avoid** are those added to foods that have little or no other nutritional value, and as I said, if you do no more than cut these down to a bare minimum, it will do absolute wonders for your skin.

In summary here, to deprive your body of fruit is to deprive it of one of the best and most potent sources of anti-oxidants and other nutrients that nature offers and this is why you will often find its inclusion in my serving ideas and recommended recipes. However do be sensible over the amounts you eat and see it as part of an overall balanced diet, rather than a green light for you to eat as much as you want. Be sparing with dried fruit which, although nutritious, is very "moreish" and can fuel the sugar cravings that you are trying to eradicate.

Excess Salt

As previously mentioned, salt is vital to life and to attempt to completely eliminate it from your diet can be dangerous and result in a deficiency of essential minerals, apart from the fact that for many people their food will seem dull and uninteresting.

1. At home, what you need to do is to **substitute unrefined salt for refined salt.** Unrefined salt is simply bursting with more than 60 essential and nourishing minerals which will a) help prevent or correct dehydration and reduce fluid retention for a taut and luminous skin b) encourage the healthy maintenance and renewal of your skin's cells c) promote an improved absorption of nutrients in your gastro-intestinal tract, and d) promote a healthy immune system to protect your skin from infections and disease

2. Your body will find it **easier to absorb and process** salt that is as close to its natural state as possible, and although the sodium content will be the same you will probably find that you need to use less on and in your food because

of the resulting purity of the taste. I actually find the taste of refined salt really "thin" in comparison.

3. Be careful of **misleading labeling** - anything called simply "sea salt", even when purchased from a natural health store – is almost always refined. The label should specifically state that the product is "unrefined" to avoid any possible misunderstanding, as this is yet another way in which consumers are grossly mislead.

4. For your everyday needs you can't do better than *Redmond Sea Salt* which is also available in a more finely ground formula if that is what you prefer (I personally just put unrefined salt crystals into my regular salt grinder). Another brand you might consider is *Celtic Sea Salt* which is particularly good in bringing out the flavour of meat, however this is quite a bit more expensive than the Redmond brand. Both are available online and in some health stores.

5. I have also recently seen on the supermarket shelves, although have yet to try, an organically approved *Atlantic Sea Salt* by a company called Geo-Organics. This appears to be a 100% sustainable product that involves no chemical processing.

6. Acquire the habit of **adding less salt** when cooking, and at the table. Always taste your

food first to see if it genuinely needs extra seasoning. Be aware also, that the hungrier you are the more salt you'll be tempted to add.

7. Try experimenting with **alternative seasonings** such as ground black pepper, herbs, garlic or lemon/lime juice. These can be added to almost any meat or vegetable dish. Spices such as turmeric, cumin or paprika add a wonderful dimension to many pastas or stews, and stir-fries are instantly "lifted" by the addition of ginger, chilli, lime-juice and garlic.

All of the above have wonderful health-giving properties in their own right – for example turmeric and ginger both have anti-inflammatory properties which can particularly benefit your heart. Ginger is also great to help keep your circulation in tip-top condition due to its supply of calcium, magnesium, phosphorus and potassium.

8. Rather than buying cooking sauces that are often high in salt, **make your own sauce** using ripe and flavoursome tomatoes, onions, a touch of garlic or herbs, chopped olives, a squeeze of lime juice etc. Any surplus can be frozen and stored.

9. **Be careful when buying gravy and stock** as many of these products are high in salt. Either look out for low-salt alternatives, or experiment

in making your own which, as with cooking sauces, can be frozen and stored.

10. **Roast or bake vegetables** such as tomatoes and red peppers, courgettes, parsnips, carrots, squashes, or fennel. This method of cooking brings out the lovely flavour of the vegetables so lessening the need to drown them in salt.

11. **Avoid crisps and salted nuts**, substituting unsalted nuts, fruit, or vegetable "sticks" instead. Remember that the salt added to these snacks will invariably be heavily processed, and as such very damaging to your health and to your skin.

12. Also **reduce your intake of known salty products** like cheese and bacon (try reduced-salt, unsmoked back bacon), canned or packet soups, soy sauce, baked beans, mustard, pickles, salad dressings, stocks, cured or smoked meats, fast–food sandwiches, most breakfast cereals, and all processed ready meals (especially low fat versions) and takeaways.

13. As with sugar, start to look around for **brands with a lower salt content,** brands such as **Sanchi**, a premium range of Japanese sauces, condiments and oils that also combine well with western foods.

Sanchi pride themselves on their range of whole and natural foods using sustainable, quality ingredients such as natural and unrefined sea salt. Their products have no additives or preservatives, minimal sugar content and absolutely no GM ingredients, and 40% of their range is organic.

○ Try **Sanchi organic shoyu soy sauce**, aged for 18 months in cedar wood barrels and ideal as a savoury seasoning in place of salt. Add just before the end of cooking, to soups and stocks, marinades, sauces, stir fries or any vegetable or fish dish. If you are wheat intolerant then try their gluten-free **tamari soy sauce** which has a slightly richer taste than the Shoyu.

These products can be found in most health food and organic stores and in some supermarkets. Alternatively purchase online for home delivery at www.goodfooddelivery.co.uk or telephone direct on 02476 541990.

○ Try **Kikkoman** products too, their low-salt soy sauce contains only 3.62g of salt per every 100ml of sauce, with no fat and only 3.9gm sugar. Compare this to the well known leading brand *Amoy* whose corresponding product still contains a whopping (in comparison) 11.3g per 100ml, not to mention 9.2gm sugar, additional colour, preservative, and flavour enhancers (E631 and E627). Both products taste great, the choice is yours to make!

There are healthy alternatives for most products nowadays if you look for them, the problem is that the vast majority of people are so conditioned to buying higher profile and mass-produced brands that they are unaware of, or unwilling to recognize, the need for change.

Remember that even within your regular "supermarket" brands there will be varying amounts of salt which leads me on to my next point:

14. **Read the nutritional labels!** As a rule, a high salt content is 1.5g (0.6g of sodium) or more per 100g, and a low salt content is 0.3g (0.1g of sodium) or less per 100g. As with fat and sugar levels, if colour coding is used then RED = High, AMBER = Medium and GREEN = Low. Compare the labels on all foods you buy, and opt for those that have less or no added salt.

15. Be aware that **"no added salt" or "unsalted" does not necessarily mean that the product is entirely salt-free**, as there could be natural sodium already present in the food. However I would urge you to become aware of the huge amounts of *the wrong sort of hidden salt* that you consume in a day, and adjust your

shopping habits accordingly. Become an expert even, and use your knowledge to educate family and friends - and remember to substitute a good quality unrefined salt, in small amounts, for use at home.

16. Interestingly, **"no salt" foods usually contain less suga**r (craftily added to regular products by our trusty manufacturers to counterbalance the salt). So by opting for low salt or unsalted products you will kill two birds with one stone so to speak.

17. The message here is low salt not no salt so follow these steps for yet another piece in place in the jigsaw and in the full picture that is of a skin repaired and restored from inside out.

Wheat and AGEs

As mentioned earlier, this is a bit of a grey area for me, because although research has thrown up hard evidence as to the potential ageing effects of wheat, wholewheat products are so highly nutritious I would hesitate to suggest eliminating them from your diet altogether.

Wheat germ supplement, in my opinion, is so jam-packed with vital nutrients as to be called a "miracle food" and I have used this regularly for many years. However if you are a wheat tolerant person yet want to cut down your intake of wheat products due to their associated effects on ageing, then here are one or two suggested alternatives:

1. Use **Spelt flour** in any recipe that calls for wheat flour. It is a low AGE carbohydrate that is ideal for hand baking and additionally has a lower gluten content. It is also highly nutritious, being an excellent source of magnesium, manganese, iron, B complex vitamins and fibre.

   Look for it in health food stores and delicatessens, farm shops and garden centres. Some supermarkets such as Waitrose stock organic white and whole grain spelt flour. Its only downside is that it doesn't work so well in bread making machines.

2. Another alternative to wheat flour is **buckwheat flour.** This has a deliciously rich nutty flavour and, like spelt flour, is extremely nutritious, being an excellent source of fibre, protein, amino acids, B vitamins and magnesium.

   Buckwheat also boasts a rich supply of some particular flavonoids/phyto nutrients that act as anti-oxidants, working with the magnesium to relax blood vessels and improve the transportation of nutrients through a more efficient circulatory system. These compounds may also be instrumental in controlling blood sugar levels.

In addition to all of the above, buckwheat flour is gluten-free (make sure that this is specifically stated on the label, as it can sometimes be blended with wheat as a filler). Its rich nuttiness makes it a very delicious ingredient in cakes, puddings and pancakes but like spelt it does not work so well for bread making as it can affect the performance of the dough. If you like the flavour and want to use it to make bread, then combine it with a regular whole-wheat flour in a 50/50 mix.

3. Experiment also, with other wheat-free grains such as **rye** which provide an interesting and different taste experience to tickle your taste buds!

4. If you still prefer your regular wheat flour then **opt for a natural whole-grain** type that has not been heavily processed and lost all its beneficial oils and nutritional content. As with spelt flour you can find it in health food stores, most supermarkets, delicatessens, farm shops and garden centres (the Wessex Mill brand offers a very good range of products and is widely available).Processed white flour, like processed salt, has been chemically altered for four main reasons:

   ○ it looks more appealing

   ○ it has a lighter texture that is easier to use

○ it lasts longer on your kitchen shelf and

○ it is therefore more profitable to the manufacturers. And it has absolutely no goodness in it whatsoever …

5. **Bake your own bread!** There's no need to spend a massive amount of money in order to fill your kitchen with the delicious smell of baking, even if you need to invest in a bread maker. I picked one up from the local bargain pages for under £15 ten years ago, and it is still going strong! Check out eBay also, to broaden your choice still further.

6. Alternatively, if you really don't have time, or the inclination to do your own baking, then while you're out and about be on the look-out for **small local bakeries** that use natural ingredients and with no additives in their products.

   Only last week, in a small town about eight miles from where I live, I found a local bakery selling the most delicious loaves - baked on the premises from 100% natural and unrefined ingredients, with no additives or preservatives and with gluten-free options to boot. It is these little niche businesses that you need to develop a nose for. It doesn't matter if they are not local, you can buy a stache of loaves and freeze them.

7. If neither of these options suits you for whatever reason, then just **buy the best whole grain and organic loaves** you can find on the supermarket shelf.

   Whichever options you choose, if wheat flour is an ingredient then moderate your intake for reasons previously mentioned. However I do believe wheat to be a very staple and nutritious part of a balanced diet, and one that offers significant health benefits.

8. With regard to **reducing the amount of AGEs** produced in your body generally, then there are two things you need to do … *firstly* cut down on your consumption of those foods known to contain high levels of AGEs such as red meat, dairy produce, products made from regular wheat flour, and all smoked or processed foods … and *secondly*, avoid on a regular basis any cooking methods using a high heat that causes browning (or worse still, blackening) of your food, opting instead for steaming, poaching or boiling, and making lots of easy and delicious one-pot meals such as casseroles or curries (a slow cooker is ideal for this purpose).

   o Swap your morning toast for a dish of creamy quinoa porridge made with almond or coconut milk (cooking time around 15mns) with a sprinkling of berries for anti-oxidant content, or alternatively some poached or scrambled eggs with a slice of nutritious spelt or wholemeal bread.

○ If you can't give up toast completely, then try at least to only lightly brown it - and substitute a different breakfast on alternate days. Remember, this plan is all about making informed and healthy changes to your lifestyle *that are sustainable* in the long-term …

○ You should also make a habit of adding spices such as cinnamon, ginger, turmeric and cumin to your food while cooking. In addition to numerous other health benefits, these will all protect against the formation of AGEs – as will apple cider vinegar which works by lowering blood sugar levels. Dilute about a tablespoon in a small amount of water before adding to any dish. Lemon or lime juice also works well for this purpose due to its acidic properties.

Toxins, Chemicals and Synthetic Oils

Yet again, a huge topic to cover and without turning this little book into something akin to War and Peace, there is not enough space to go into it in great depth. However I have listed what I hope to be some actionable ways in which you can reduce your daily exposure to these dastardly enemies of your health and, ultimately, of your skin.

174

1. If you are a smoker, then **Stop Smoking**! This will rid your body of one of the greatest toxic overloads it will ever encounter. Refer back to the beginning of this chapter for more suggestions on how to go about this.

   Without meaning to sound harsh, if you are not prepared to make the attempt to at least drastically cut down on your daily quota of cigarettes then you shouldn't really be reading this book. If you want to keep your health, your looks and your lovely skin then you need to give up – there is no easy way to say it…you can't have it both ways

2. Refer back to the earlier section on toxins and chemicals, then start by scrutinising the labels on every cleaning product you buy.

   Although manufacturers are not obliged to list all of the active ingredients, the levels of toxicity are often indicated by such words as **danger**, **poison**, **warning** or **caution** with *danger* and *poison* indicating the most dangerous in terms of toxicity, *caution* indicating the least dangerous, although still carrying a significant risk factor, and *warning* somewhere between the two. This is usually followed by a more specific warning which alerts you to the exact nature of the risk you take in using the product: for example "may cause skin irritation", "avoid contact with eyes and skin", "corrosive", or "extremely flammable".

I have in front of me a common branded mould and mildew remover in aerosol spray formulation, which actually gives very specific health warnings about its contents:

○ Under "directions for use" and "uses" on the back label (many people never actually get beyond this point) it displays a clearly visible red strip with the word "Cautions" in white lettering. Underneath this, it tells you that the product contains sodium hypochlorite and to "Keep out of sight and reach of children and pets".

○ It also tells you that "this product is [note: not "can be" but "is"] irritating to eyes and skin. Avoid contact with skin and eyes…in case of contact with eyes rinse immediately with plenty of water and seek medical advice…if swallowed, seek medical advice immediately and show this container or label…do not breathe spray…as with any household product avoid prolonged skin contact with this product…for sensitive skin the use of gloves is recommended…wash and dry hands after use…do not use with other products…may release dangerous gases (chlorine).

○ Just in case you still haven't got the message, there is also a large black cross in a bright orange box with **"irritant"** printed below!

The dangers are clear so **why** do people continue to buy this and other similar products?

Well the answer is firstly that these products are all common place on the shelves and are relatively cheap to buy (many can be bought for a pound or less at Poundland or Home Bargains), and secondly that many people only glance at the label to check the product is right for whatever it is they want it for, and that it is quick and easy to use. Beyond that I genuinely don't think they are particularly interested in what they see as "small print", and I totally get this as when in a hurry and faced with a lot of reading or a haze of scientific-sounding words, my eyes definitely have the tendency to glaze over.

If people do afford the warnings a second glance then the feeling is either, "Oh well, it must be alright or they wouldn't be allowed to sell it" or "Well of course they have to print this to cover themselves, and everyone else is using it so I'm sure it's ok." However **you** now know better and so are in a strong position to make informed choices.

To this end avoid all such products. Also, if any active ingredients are listed, give a particularly wide berth to those that contain **ammonia** or **chlorine**. As I say, you would be amazed at how many of the general public never, ever, look at what's in the product they are buying or if they do, they don't fully understand the risks so just buy it anyway. Manufacturers rely on this fact to sell their products. And just so you remain focused, do remember the message at the heart of this book, that when your health is compromised in any way then the effect will be seen or felt, sooner or later, in your skin.

3. Be wary of any household products that include the word **fragrance** in their labeling. This refers in particular to products such as fabric conditioners and air fresheners in which the added fragrance, lovely though it may be to use, can cause significant allergic reactions from the respiratory system, eyes and skin in certain people.

4. Beware too, of personal care products. That cloud of perfume -however expensive - that you so lavishly spray around your neck, décolletage and pulse points, is awash with chemicals just waiting to be inhaled, as are any of your body-care products containing added fragrance such as deodorants, hair and body sprays and many items of make-up.

Avoid wherever possible, and start looking around instead for less harmful alternatives containing mostly natural and plant-based ingredients. There are some lovely natural perfume oils produced from plants that smell divine and will not harm you, and many good ranges of personal care products and make-up using natural fragrance, available in some stores and online.

Try your local health stores such as **Holland & Barrett.** I particularly like their **Dr Organic** range) or look online for smaller niche companies selling a vast array of naturally derived products using, for example, a*loe vera, jojoba, vitamin E, coconut oil* and *almond oil*.

All of this is yet another area where you may find it easier to work on a "gradual replacement" basis ... as one of your regular products comes to an end then simply replace it with a less toxic and more eco-friendly alternative.

5. If you cannot avoid using any of these toxic products, then please do take the warnings on the labels very seriously. Do not inhale the spray from an aerosol, as the droplets will find their way straight into your lungs. If you can, hold something over your mouth and nose and do not remain in the area where you have sprayed, any longer than is necessary.

Beware too, of areas of broken skin and do not allow them to come into contact with any wipes, liquids or sprays containing toxic substances.

6. Be on the lookout for any **signs of localized irritation** such as rashes, pustules etc, which are indications of blocked pores and a stressed skin. *You may not have had any bad reactions in the past, but this does not automatically guarantee that you will not have a reaction of some kind in the future.* As you may remember in Part One, I mentioned that as you get older the balance of bacteria existing naturally on your skin can change with decreasing levels of oestrogen, and this does mean that your skin will react differently with various elements and ingredients, to how it did when you were younger.

7. Try to use more **eco-friendly cleaners** that are so much better for your health and the environment. You may find some in the larger supermarkets or hardware stores, but many are still only available in health food stores, online or through catalogues. Brands such as *Ecover, Kleeneze, BioShield* and *Earth Friendly* offer the consumer environmentally friendly alternatives that, although not totally harmless in my opinion, will not so drastically compromise your health or the integrity of your skin.

An added bonus is that by using these products you will also be creating a safer environment for other members of your household, especially elderly people, children and pets. The major drawback is that they are more expensive than standard "off the shelf" products, so if you are on a budget then skip to No.8 below.

8. Alternatively you can **change to using simple, cheaper and time-tested ingredients** that will clean your house just as well, and in some cases better, than their more modern counterparts -ingredients such as soap and water, vinegar, lemon juice, baking soda and borax.

   o **Baking soda** works a treat in bathrooms for removing lime-scale and mould, and in kitchens as a natural all-purpose cleaner. It can either be mixed to a paste with some water, or simply sprinkled onto a wet sponge or cloth to clean bathtubs and sinks, countertops, ovens etc.

   o **Borax** is also tough on mould, the only drawback being that it is toxic *if consumed* so keep out of the reach of children and pets.

   o **Lemon juice** is the most deliciously-smelling, non-toxic substitute for bleach, and can be mixed with baking soda to deal with stubborn stains or simply when scrubbing over surfaces in the kitchen or bathroom. It also makes a good fabric stain-remover, and can be added to laundry during the rinse cycle.

o Last, but by no means least, **Vinegar** is such a fantastically versatile product that whole books have been written to extol its virtues! Simply mix equal parts of vinegar and water to effectively and safely clean practically any surface in your house. It will cut through grease and can be used neat in sinks or in the toilet bowl, or to clean windows.

o An added bonus to those people who dislike *spiders* in their house (very like myself!) is that spiders hate the smell of both lemon and vinegar, and the regular use of either or both will keep your home a fresh-smelling and relatively spider-free zone!

9. Try to **remove the need for harsh drain cleaners** by doing what you can to prevent sinks and drains from becoming blocked in the first place (always good practice in any household).

For instance if you have a large pan of greasy water, empty it down the toilet rather than your kitchen sink. **Avoid** letting scraps of food escape down the sink when you are washing up by making sure you scrape any residue into the bin before washing, and by using a little plastic or metal drain screen, which can be purchased cheaply from any home or hardware store. Use one in the bathroom to trap hair and prevent it from clogging up plug holes.

These simple measures will prevent most simple blockages but if you are unlucky enough to get one then **invest in a plunger**, a wonderful and relatively inexpensive contraption that will remove the blockage by suction.

10. **Do not use antibacterial products** as prolonged use will eventually result in the creation of antibiotic-resistant bacteria. This is why doctors are now so reluctant to prescribe antibiotics for coughs and sore throats. You can clean just as effectively using any of the natural products listed above.

11. To **reduce your exposure to BPAs** (as discussed in Section One) avoid microwaving food in plastic containers. If you cannot avoid buying processed meals then at least transfer the food onto a microwaveable plate and wrap round with a piece of kitchen towel to cover instead. In the case of soups and other liquids, pour them into a saucepan and heat on the hob.

Buy fresh food wherever possible and opt for non plastic containers to store it in such as stainless steel, glass or ceramic. Best of all, replace existing plastic containers with BPA free alternatives.

Some of the larger garden centres such as Webbs stock a large range of plastic-type BPA free products, including lunch boxes, storage containers for cereals etc., jugs for water or juice, soup mugs and water bottles. I am told there is a large market for these products, so it would appear that people are finally becoming more aware of, and expressing concern over, this issue. Your food can so easily be contaminated by what you store or cook it in and this is something you should be aware of.

To the same end, when buying saucepans, frying pans or other cookware, always invest in the best you can afford so that you don't end up with half the metal lining of the pan in your food - and always use a **wooden spoon**.

One last point about BPAs is that they are also apparently contained in thermal, or carbonless, till receipts so remember to wash your hands well after handling these.

12. Finally, with regard to any skin-care products you have been accustomed to using, as part of your transition to a holistic method of skin care

then opt for those that contain **plant-based oils** such as almond, jojoba, aloe-vera or pure coconut which are more easily absorbed and support your skin from the inside.

Petroleum-based oils are known to be carcinogenic, and *mineral oils* are comedogenic which means that they will block your pores and not allow your skin to breathe. The end result of this will be blackheads, spots and pimples. Look for products that have the fewest - and the purest - ingredients, and avoid any containing ingredients that you do not recognize or cannot pronounce.

My point here is that it seems crazy to spend a lot of money on a product containing, for example, vitamin E "**as one ingredient**" amongst all manner of other added stuff that is harmful to your skin, when you can buy vitamin E oil on its own, in its purest and most natural form and free from all chemicals and preservatives that can seriously compromise its wonderful benefits. Be Brave…Ditch your regular skin cream and I promise you your skin will not suffer in the slightest.

Pesticides and Other Chemicals in your food

It can be difficult to eradicate this risk from your lifestyle as the alternatives are either time consuming, or too expensive for many people. However it is worth considering the following options, remembering that any changes - however small – are better than to make no changes at all.

1. **Thoroughly wash** all fruits, vegetables, salad items and rice before consuming. Washing does not guarantee the removal of all traces of pesticide, but it may remove some. I have also read that gently scrubbing your vegetables with a few drops of vinegar in the water can offer extra protection.

2. Buy **fresh, local and organic produce** whenever you can, particularly meat products such as chicken, turkey and ham. Many farm shops now have a tea-room and gift store, so you can turn this into a lovely family outing each weekend, maybe combining it with a country ramble afterwards.

   Note: Without any doubt at all, "*Fresh is Best*" – BUT, in the case of fruit and vegetables, it really needs to be produce that you have grown yourself or have bought from a local source such as a farm shop and that still retains its full quota of nutrients.

   o The problem with, for instance fresh vegetables bought from the supermarket or other high-street shops, is that they are purposely picked before fully ripened in order to preserve their shelf life, and this means that their nutritional content is not at its peak. Further nutrients are then lost in transportation, and by the time they've also spent several days on the supermarket shelf, then even more in your fridge, there is very little goodness left in them.

o   In this instance I would say reluctantly that you are better off buying canned or frozen, as although the freezing and canning processes destroy certain nutrients the vegetables are in peak condition when picked and are then frozen/canned very quickly, thus sealing in all remaining nutrients. Be aware that some brands add extra sugar and salt to canned products, so make sure you check for this before buying.

3. **When eating out** look for places that use organic and preferably free range food. I am lucky in having a small deli with a tea room near to where I live, that sells and cooks only organic and free range food – dishes such as eggs on rye bread with mushrooms, mushrooms fried in organic olive oil with garlic and blue cheese piled onto home-baked bread, organic burgers, and a choice of several delicious meals.

Obviously it will not always be possible to do this as niche eating places of this kind are, relatively speaking, in the minority. However if there is a choice available to you then make use of it.

4. When buying packaged foods be on the look-out for those using **organic ingredients** and try to avoid any that use artificial colourings or dyes, additives such as monosodium glutamate (MSG), artificial sweeteners like aspartame or saccharin, and preservatives. Any packaged food that contains either "E" numbers or any listed ingredient you can't pronounce, by very virtue of this fact contains a level of toxins that are potentially harmful when ingested over a lifetime.

5. Aim to *gradually replace* all of your refined, processed and oh, so unhealthy foodstuffs (for example, flour, sugar rice, salt and stocks) with whole and unrefined alternatives that have not had all the goodness stripped from them and are not pumped full of chemical preservatives, flour improvers, acidity regulators and the like. *If you buy a bag of wholewheat flour then "wholewheat flour" should really be the only listed ingredient.*

6. Try to **avoid microwaving food in plastic containers** as this process will just add to any toxins already present in the food. Microwaving in itself of course, is also considered hazardous to health, but understandably many people would be lost without the convenience of a microwave so

just try to use other methods of cooking or heating food whenever you can. In other words, use if you need to but avoid where possible.

7. **Bake your own bread**, using unrefined flour that has no added chemicals (see previous section on wheat). Or buy organic bread made from unprocessed ingredients that are actually *good* for you.

8. **Fit a filter** to your tap or drink bottled water. Tap water, although like everything else not noticeably hazardous in the short term, contains chlorine, fluoride, heavy metals and other contaminants, all of which are toxic to your health. Think about it for a moment … all these substances are added to our water in order to kill bacteria and other hazardous compounds so it stands to reason that they must be strong stuff and not really a good idea to deliberately allow your body exposure to.

9. And finally, if the subject of pesticides on your food is of serious concern to you, then hire an allotment and start to **grow your own fruit and veg.** All the healthy exercise and fresh air, plus the luxury of eating completely natural and chemical-free food, will not only be rewarding but will have inestimable benefits on your health. Plus you can always sell, or give to grateful friends, all the surplus vegetables that you are unable to use yourself!

Note: with regard to everything you have read so far in this section, pass the time while you're next waiting in the queue at the supermarket by thinking about all the things that are "wrong" with the contents of the person's trolley in front of you … this can prove to be quite an enlightening and empowering – not to mention entertaining - exercise!

Air Pollution

You can reduce your exposure to air pollutants in the following ways:

1. When exercising out of doors in urban areas, try to **avoid areas of heavy traffic**, opting instead for quieter back-streets or parks. Avoid the kerb side of the pavement also, as the air here will contain higher levels of particulates.

2. **Work out in the early morning or late evening** if possible, as fumes from both traffic and the ozone will be at their lowest at these times.

3. If you are passed by any vehicle emitting thick, black fumes then make a conscious effort **not to inhale** them. Hold a hanky over your nose and mouth, or at the very least turn your head away and shallow-breathe until you are well clear of the area.

4. Check out the new **smart phone App** that has been developed to help you identify and avoid polluted areas. Search for "city air" at "itunes.apple.com".

5. If **traveling by bus** avoid sitting next to the engine (upper deck is best).

6. **Cleanse** your skin thoroughly after exposure.

7. Indoors, make sure you **have your boilers, heaters and chimneys** (if you have them) **inspected on a regular basis**.

8. Use a **dehumidifier** to effectively reduce humidity levels and discourage mould.

9. Ensure your rooms are **adequately ventilated** at all times as it is important that the air should not be allowed to remain static. Make sure your air is refreshed at least once a day and most particularly if you or anyone in the household has a cold or cough. Sitting around breathing in your own or somebody else's germs is the surest way to pass around, or to prolong, an infection.

10. As discussed in the previous section, **cut down on your use of toxic household products** and consider the use of natural alternatives. Dispose properly of old paints and varnishes, and do not leave them standing

around once finished with, to release their toxic compounds into the air you breathe.

11. Finally, **be aware of cold, flu and vomiting bugs that may be airborne,** as repeated infections spell disaster for the appearance and vitality of your skin and cold sores can actually leave permanent damage in the worst case scenario. So do your bit to help prevent the spread of infection by always using tissues (which should be properly disposed of after use, preferably by flushing down a toilet) and regularly wiping all hard surfaces in the home including door handles and light switches.

If you touch handles or handrails while you are out, then make sure your hands are properly washed (just flipped back into "nurse-mode" here!). At the very least use an antiseptic gel, if you have no access to washing facilities, before eating or putting your hands near your face and mouth (I carry a small bottle of it in my handbag at all times).

With the right knowledge and by exercising proper care, it should be possible to drastically reduce the risk both of catching or spreading a cold. Prevention is, as always, a far better option than the alternative.

Most of these suggestions are good general housekeeping practice anyway, but with a little care and thought you can remove a lot of potential threats that can damage your health and the appearance and integrity of your skin.

Weight Loss

I'm not actually going to spend a huge amount of time on this subject as it is such a massive issue in its own right, and this is not so much my area of expertise. Also I imagine that many readers who wish to lose weight for whatever reason, will already be involved in a weight loss plan that suits them or be registered with Weight Watchers, Slimming World or similar organizations.

I *will* say again, however, that a slow and steady weight-loss plan is the only way to go if you want to preserve your looks and the integrity of your skin, so to this end:

1. **Avoid any form of fast weight loss** or yo-yo dieting.

2. For the purpose of preserving your youthful looks while losing weight, **avoid low-fat diets**. You know now that low-fat foods contain extra sugar which, apart from being a killer for your skin, converts into fat in the long-run anyway - so where's the point in this? By very virtue of the fact that they are low-fat, these foods are also most often high in carbohydrates, so you will end up with a double whammy of sugar content.

In addition to this, as I mentioned earlier, anything advertised as low-fat is not a "real" or whole food and has few, if any, benefits for your health.

3. If you would like to lose weight but are not currently on any sort of diet, then to **action the advice in this book** will almost certainly result in an incidental weight loss as your body becomes used to its new, healthier regime. Not only will your diet be full of delicious, health-promoting foods, but your entire system will start to function more efficiently and be better able to process and assimilate the various nutrients for transportation around your body. Simply cut out all processed, fatty and sugary foods from your diet to lose up to half a stone in no time at all!

To sum up, too much excess weight is bad for your body on many levels as it will, at some point in your life, result in serious health issues that will greatly impact on the ageing process and on your skin. So yes, to lose weight is good, however fast weight loss is *not* good as you will risk ending up with wrinkly, saggy skin that is unattractive and extremely ageing. **Opt for a nice, slow and steady weight loss that you can maintain for life** - your body and your skin will love you for it!

Lack of Exercise

Regular exercise is **vital to the functioning of every system in your body**. It increases your heart rate thereby increasing the blood flow that carries oxygen and nutrients to your cells and vital organs, and it assists in the removal of waste products, including free radicals, from your cells. It is also a great stress-buster, a very important benefit as stress can have serious repercussions on the health and appearance of your skin and will improve both your body image and self-esteem.

1. If you do not engage in any form of physical exercise then you first need to **identify the reasons why.** The most common reasons are "I don't have time", "I'm too tired" or "I don't have the money to spend on exercise classes or the gym". Once you have acknowledged these reasons, said them "out loud" as it were, then you are in a better position to find ways round these stumbling blocks in your mind.

2. Firstly, the words **exercise** and **gym** do not necessarily belong in the same sentence. Going to the gym is not compulsory and is certainly not the only way to increase the amount of exercise you do. Yes, it is a great way to exercise your larger muscles, to improve your level of fitness and to generally tone up your body - and if two or three concentrated sessions a week could work for you then bite the bullet and go for it.

Private gym membership is expensive, but most **local councils** have facilities that are far more reasonably priced and with concessions for those on low incomes or at certain times of day, so ask around.

3. Once again, motivate yourself by using the **visualization technique:** imagine how you will look after even three months of gym training and let that thought drive you forward. Alternatively think of someone you admire and would love to look like and keep that vision in mind while you train.

4. Just be aware that excessive and strenuous cardiac exercise can cause oxidative stress in healthy skin cells, which is a primary cause of ageing skin and wrinkles. Combat this by cleansing your skin thoroughly before and after your workout, keeping it well hydrated both internally (via your anti-oxidant and fluid intake) and externally with a hydrating spray.

5. If the gym doesn't grab you then explore other forms of exercise that increase your heart rate and tone your large muscle groups, exercise such as **fast walking, cycling, swimming, dancing,** or, with reservations as it can be damaging for your joints, **jogging**.

Most of these activities can be enjoyed either alone, if you prefer, or in company as part of a sociable time spent with (old or new) friends.

Look out for what is currently available in your area, not only in the way of facilities such as leisure centres or tennis courts, but organized activities like nature rambles that are both healthy, fun and educational for the whole family

6. **Incorporate** exercise into your daily routine with very little extra effort and without taking too much time out of your busy day:

   o Always **use the stairs instead of the lift**, running up them as quickly as you can (this always looks and feels impressive!).

   o Whenever you have the time, **walk instead of taking the car** (to the shops, the library, taking the children to school etc.).

   o If you work try to **make time in your lunch break for a brisk walk** around the block or round a nearby park, if there is one, especially if your job is a sedentary one. Not only will this get your circulation moving again but it will blow away the cobwebs, recharge your brain-power and help disperse the morning's stress.

   o If you work in the city then make sure you take steps to avoid as many of the traffic fumes as you can, as outlined in the section on air pollution. On balance the exercise will still do you more good than sitting at the same desk, in the same office, breathing in the same air that you have been doing all morning!

○ Most **household chores** involve a degree of fairly strenuous exercise, so do exploit this for all it's worth! Put on some upbeat music while you work, to encourage you to get into a rhythm and make the most of any opportunities to bend, stretch, or work up a sweat. Seasonal activities such as sweeping away leaves or shoveling snow are excellent for increasing your heart-rate and toning your muscles.

7. When deciding on **family days out**, go for anything that involves lots of walking. Theme parks and wildlife centres, arboretums, national trust, woodland, local hills, parks or the beach (if you live near any of these) are great choices to make and do not all involve spending a lot of money. Take a picnic if the weather's fine, so you don't need to spend money buying over-priced food.

8. Children and dogs in particular, are some of the best excuses you can have to get out there in the fresh air and exercise. Walk with them, play with them and chase them around, anything to get those muscles working and the blood pumping.

9. For best results you do need to **exercise at least 3 times a week for around 20 minutes**, very gradually increasing this time to half an hour as your body adjusts to its new routine. Ensure that you always warm up before more strenuous activities (such as dancing, tennis or a workout) with some gentle stretching - and that afterwards you spend five minutes or so to stretch your muscles out again and allow your heart rate to return to normal.

Stress

Stress is the latest thing to make headlines in the beauty industry as having a significant effect on the ageing process and when you consider both the mental and physical traumas that it causes your body, this actually makes perfect sense.

Like most of us I've had a fair amount of stress in my life. I remember times when I've had so many things to think of that my mind has been like a roundabout that wouldn't stop. I was completely incapable of isolating any one thing to actually focus on or try to deal with. This was really frustrating, as some really vitally important tasks took me two to three weeks to get round to doing, yet once I'd finally managed to focus my mind only actually took around ten minutes to complete.

Out of all the following ways therefore, that may help in coping with stress levels, my number one priority is this:

1. **Take up the reins again and take control of your life. Nothing, but nothing, is more empowering**:

   o Find yourself a piece of paper and a pen and make a list - it doesn't matter how long - of all the things you need to deal with or attend to. Even the sheer effort of writing out that list will make you feel better straight away.

   o Once you have done this then you need to prioritize these tasks so that you can systematically start at the top and focus exclusively on that one thing until it is completed. At this point you draw a very satisfying line through it and move on to the next. I cannot tell you how good this makes you feel, and what a positive effect it will have on your state of mind.

   o Once you have worked your way through everything on your list, then try to continue with this practice on a day-to-day basis. It will help you pinpoint what you want to achieve within a certain time-frame, and instill in you the discipline that you need in order to actually focus on doing it.

   o If there are any tasks about which you are particularly concerned or anxious (all those "sleepless nights" sort of tasks) then try to tackle them first thing in the morning while you are fresh and your mind is uncluttered, rather than to keep putting them off, as this only serves to increase your stress levels and achieves absolutely nothing in either the short or the long-term.

2. **If you are a "bottler"** who finds it difficult to talk about your problems to others, then try opening up to just one friend or family member who you feel would understand, or ideally someone who is going through a similar thing to yourself. If you are really not comfortable with this then there are many advisory or support groups out there (depending on what it is you are worried about) to help. You can find these on the internet or in places like your local library or Citizen's Advice - or ask your GP.

3. **If your stress is due to pressure of work**, then you need to learn how to say "no" sometimes if the demands of your employer are unreasonable. Try to do this tactfully and have some alternative suggestions at hand for consideration, as to how the extra workload could be better managed or shared out.

If you work for yourself then perhaps you need to learn how to delegate more, or simply take on less work. If your business is flagging and this is not possible, then you urgently need to take professional advice as to the best way forward as you will add years to your biological age through overwork, worry, lack of sleep and not eating proper meals (all of which are by-products of stress) and the problems will still be there at the end of the day.

Problems with your business do not necessarily mean you will have to close down but you may need help in deciding the best way forward, even if this means completely re-branding the whole caboodle. Just talking things through and throwing around a few suggestions with someone who is there to help, will do a lot to relieve pent up stress - but *you* are the one who has to make this happen and sooner rather than later.

4. Even on a personal level, for example **pressure from family or friends** to frequently help them out or accept invitations that you are too busy, or cannot afford, to accept, then you need to be able to firmly but pleasantly say "no" on occasion. No-one need be hurt or offended by this, especially if you always have an alternative proposition to hand:

For instance you could say something like "I'm really sorry I'm not able to go for coffee with you tomorrow as I've rather a lot on at the moment, but perhaps I could call you when things have calmed down a bit and we could make another date when we're both free?". Just make sure that the negative ("I'm really sorry but I can't ...") is followed immediately by a positive ("...but perhaps we could ..."), and you should have no problems. Make sure though, that you do actually follow through with what you promised, otherwise it will carry no credence in the future and friends will very soon become disenchanted with you!

5. Always aim to **put aside some time each day** that is just for your own relaxation and the things you enjoy doing: things like taking time out for a long, scented bath or shower and pampering session, cooking yourself a proper, nourishing meal, reading a good book, turning down the lights and watching a good film or listening to any music that you know will put you in a good place. While you are listening, close your eyes, breathe slowly and deeply, and imagine a place where you feel happy and peaceful (a technique known as *guided imagery*, most effective when used in conjunction with relaxation or meditation CDs).

Incidentally you might like to try some **dead sea salts** in your bath, as the minerals in them work well to relax your muscles and help you de-stress. A salt bath is also wonderfully healing if you have a skin condition such as acne, eczema and psoriasis (which in itself can be very stressful). It works by a process of eliminating toxins through open pores, thereby improving circulation and decreasing inflammation. Result? Clearer, healthier skin! Highly Recommended!

6. **Exercise** is now an acknowledged stress-buster in its own right, as the increase of oxygen to your heart, lungs and brain has been proven to lessen depression and anxiety within 12 weeks. To get full benefit from this you need to do around three 20-30 minute sessions a week of any aerobic type exercise that will increase your heart rate to 120 beats per minute.

   However any form of exercise, particularly if out of doors, will help to clear your head and relieve some of the emotional stress that has accumulated over the day. Try a brisk walk, swimming, or work in the garden. Or, for sheer therapeutic value, experiment with tai chi or yoga classes which stretch out not only the body but also the mind. There's nothing like a new hobby or interest to divert your mind from your personal problems.

7. Make sure that, whatever else, you get enough **good quality sleep** as this is your body's way of restoring and repairing itself both mentally and physically. If you do not sleep properly you will have no energy and your body will run on adrenalin. Also, because sleep is a time for cell renewal, continual lack of it will leave your skin looking dull and lack-lustre. Refer to the following section on sleep for some ideas that might help your body to relax at night.

8. One of my favorite aids to relaxation (also really effective if you are trying to give up smoking, for example, or cut down on alcohol) is a wonderful, if simple, little invention called a **stress ball**. I have mentioned this before but, as repetition is the art of a good teacher, I will mention it again!

   Go to Amazon and type in "stress relievers". Your search will bring up dozens of results for stress balls in all different colours, many with cute smiley or funny faces to suit every personality, and almost all under £5! Keep one at home and/or at work and use it when you need to. Stress balls can also be helpful when you are trying to give up smoking or alcohol as they give you something to do with your hands at a time when you might be reaching for that cigarette or extra glass of wine.

9. Learn to **identify any stimulant that makes your stress worse, and AVOID**. For most people this might mean any or all of the following: alcohol, cigarettes, caffeine or sugar, most often mistakenly indulged in to relieve stress but all of which cause a temporary high followed by a crash in energy levels or mood. Plus they are addictive and they are bad for you. Smoking in particular, is now thought to be a significant cause of anxiety, stress and depression.

Instead try to find alternative ways of beating stress using some of the suggestions given above, and keep plenty of healthy snacks such as nuts, fruit or vegetable crudités on hand to nibble on.

10. Finally **avoid causing stress specifically to your skin** from external sources:

- Don't expose your skin to extreme heat or cold, or to chemicals or other irritants.

- Where you can, opt for clothing made of natural fibres, and don't wear clothes that are too tight and that risk impeding the natural flow of air around your body.

- If you get any insect bites or spots on your skin then do avoid rubbing or scratching the area. At best you will suffer unsightly skin until the sore heals, and at worst you can leave permanently damaged skin under scar tissue. Instead try a natural remedy such as **Roman chamomile oil** which, as an effective anti-inflammatory, will soothe and heal the inflamed area around your bites.

Sleep

There is nothing to match the benefits of a good night's sleep. *Lack of sleep causes bodily stress and interferes with the skin's natural ability to repair itself at night*, so in a way this section is closely linked to the previous one on stress. If you are one of those unfortunate people who find sleep difficult then you may find some of the following suggestions helpful:

1. A **regular sleeping pattern** is as important as the quality of your sleep, so try to go to bed at a similar time every night. Your body will learn through repetition when it is expected to be tired and will respond accordingly.

   To reinforce this still further, as soon as you wake up in the morning open your curtains and let the natural daylight in. This will establish your waking cycle and help keep your mind and body alert during the day, preparing your body for sleep at the expected time. If you work shifts, particularly night duty, then obviously this is not such an easy option and you will just have to try to establish the best routine you can according to the hours you work.

2. Aim for between **seven to eight hours of sleep** a night, and certainly not less than six.

3. **Anxiety and Stress** cause more sleepless nights than anything else, so with this in mind go back and re-read the previous section on stress. *Almost everything that reduces stress will also help to induce sleep*, most especially exercise. There is no substitute for either exercise or hard physical work, preferably out

of doors, as your body will become naturally and healthily tired and ready for sleep.

4. Make sure that your **mattress and pillows** are comfortable and "right" for you, especially if you have any orthopedic type problems. If this is the case you need to take advice over what would best suit your needs.

5. Always have **clean, fresh bed linen**. There is nothing like the smell and the feel of freshly laundered sheets when you climb into bed, to help you feel relaxed.

6. Make your bedroom a warm and cozy place where you want to be. Create a subtle ambience with a few simple touches like pretty scatter cushions, fresh (or even tasteful artificial) flowers, scented candles and soft lighting, all of which will help to **create a pleasurable atmosphere of warmth, relaxation and intimacy**. It goes without saying that any untidiness or clutter will have the effect of doing exactly the opposite.

Avoid also, keeping devices such as mobile phones and computers in your bedroom as it is thought that the electro-magnetic waves they emit can interfere with the quality of your sleep. Also, your bedroom should be devoid of anything that remotely smacks of work or of your busy daytime schedule.

7. If you are married or have a partner you will need to discuss how each one's nocturnal habits may affect the other - for instance if one of you wants to keep a light on and read, and the other wants the light off to go to sleep. **Understanding and compromise** is the key here, but as one person awake and tossing and turning in the night can be very disturbing for the other, any ways of improving the sleep of either partner should probably be of mutual benefit.

8. **If you are sensitive to caffeine** then it may help not to drink coffee much beyond late afternoon. Its stimulant effect can linger for several hours.

   Do have some sort of a **nightcap** though, as this is a good way to relax. A steaming hot cup of cocoa or a cup of soothing chamomile tea is really comforting and sleep inducing, even the occasional (small) glass of wine which has a calming and sedative effect in moderation.   Drink more than one glass however, and you are likely to become restless and dehydrated and this will obviously affect the quality of your sleep and the appearance of your skin when you wake up in the morning.

   A glass of freshly squeezed celery juice, sweetened if you like, with a small teaspoon of organic honey or agave nectar, is also recognized as a good natural aid to sleep.

209

9. Have a **regular soothing massage** if you can afford it or if you have a friend or partner who could do this for you - either full body or head and shoulders, and preferably just before you are ready to wind down for the evening. This will relax and de-stress your muscles and prepare your whole body for sleep.

   If you have a salon massage then opt for an aromatherapy treatment and ask your therapist to use a blend of oils known for their soothing and relaxing properties. Vigorous massages should be enjoyed at an earlier time of day as they boost the circulation and therefore have an invigorating rather than a soothing effect on your system.

10. Try sprinkling **essential oils** like *lavender* on your pillow, or dabbing a few spots on your wrists and temples. They will infuse your system with relaxing and sedative properties.

    Other essential oils that have a soporific effect and will promote sleep are c*hamomile, mandarin, jasmine, sandalwood, neroli, ylang ylang* and r*ose*. Ideally you should talk to a trained aromatherapist beforehand, who will perform a case history and recommend a blend best suited to your personal needs.

11. I would not advise sleeping tablets unless you have a deep and fundamental problem with

sleep and have tried everything else to no avail. If this is the case, then rather than the usual medication dished out by your GP try **Bach Natural Remedies Night Rescue Spray**. I have used this myself and found it to work very well. Simply apply two sprays onto your tongue just before you go to bed, close your eyes and wait for sleep.

You should have no side effects from this, and no "hung-over" feeling of drowsiness the next morning - and although it does contain a preservative and a sweetener in the base solution of malic acid, all the other ingredients are completely natural (r*ock rose, impatiens, clematis, star of Bethlehem* and *white chestnut*) to promote a deep and natural sleep.

This remedy is also available in a blister pack of *Liquid Melts* which dissolve on the tongue and are in a grape-seed oil base. Both are available from health stores such as Holland and Barrett, and larger branches of Boots.

12. Finally, try to **eat as early as you can** in the evening so your body is not still busy digesting food at bedtime, and avoid any activities that are likely to put your mind or body in a state of stress.

Chronic Pain

Chronic Pain will have devastating effects on all your bodily systems and on your skin. Apart from anything else it will tighten your muscles around the area of pain, and restrict the blood flow in that area. Your prescribed medications will also come with side effects that can bring their own health risks and can help accelerate the ageing process. Here are some suggestions that might help you relax and deal with your pain:

1. **Do not fight your pain** as this will cause stress. Instead, do your best to accept your pain and use this acceptance as a springboard to explore every possible way of dealing with it positively. Pain loves negativity and to remain hopeful and positive is one of the most effective weapons in your armoury.

2. If you have been prescribed analgesia for pain by your GP, then do not be haphazard in the way you take it. You can control the situation by **taking your medication on a regular basis** to begin with, as by doing this you are keeping your pain at a constant, subdued level.

   You need to be aware that everyone has a different pain barrier, so you cannot compare yourself to others. Waiting until the pain is so bad that you can't stand it any longer is not a good idea. Once your pain is better controlled by whatever methods you choose to use, then you can look at very gradually reducing your medication as part of a regulated plan, and with the consent of your GP.

As we looked at earlier, taking any medications long-term can have drastic side-effects, especially on your liver and kidneys - and as most tablets contain chemicals both in the coating and the ingredients used as preservatives, you do not want to take them any longer than is absolutely necessary. The same principal applies to over-the-counter medications which, due to the ease of availability, are far too widely used in my opinion.

3. Re-read the previous sections on Stress and Sleep as you need to **learn how to relax**. Discover what works best for you and practice until you can literally "switch on" as if at the touch of a button whenever you need to. Muscle tension will simply make your pain worse, and you will become tired and irritable as a result.

4. Try to **focus on the things you *are* able to enjoy**, for instance any hobbies or recreational activities you may be able to take part in, or socializing with friends. The more absorbing these activities are the better, as your involvement will take your mind off your pain.

5. Do pace yourself and learn to recognize your limits of your endurance. Take a break if you

need to - this is not giving in but rather a sign that you are in control and are dealing with your condition in a systematic and positive way.

6. **Do not hide your pain** from family and friends. Explain honestly, the problems you are experiencing and ask them if they will be encouraging and positive around you rather than just dishing out sympathy. Whilst it is good that people are sympathetic towards you, too much sympathy can be a negative reinforcement that will hinder your onwards and upwards progression. Do try though, to keep as cheerful as you can around others - as nothing will kill their goodwill more than constant misery and complaining.

7. If you feel you need more support to deal with your pain then consider asking your GP if he will refer you to a **pain clinic** where you will receive a more in-depth analysis of your problems, along with any appropriate recommendations. You could also join a local **support group** which is good in that it makes you realize you are not alone. Talking to and perhaps even helping others in a similar or worse situation than yourself is yet another way to take your mind off your own pain.

8. Explore the vast world of **alternative medicine** that offers a wide choice of holistic treatments. These could include *ayurvedic medicine,*

herbal medicine, massage and aromatherapy, acupuncture, hydrotherapy, aqua-therapy, yoga, pilates, reflexology, osteopathy and chiropractic. Certain *herbs and spices* are known to have healing properties, and this is yet another avenue you could explore.

Ask a qualified professional for advice or simply browse through your local health store and experiment to find what works for you.

Black cumin seeds for example, have been found to reduce the need for medication in some inflammatory conditions such as asthma and ulcerative colitis, although more research is needed to identify a specific therapeutic dose. Black cumin is well known for the anti-inflammatory properties of its main active ingredient **thymoquinone**, and has been used in Islamic healing for centuries. You can easily make it a part of your regular diet by simply crushing its seeds and using them in soups, curries or any dish where you want to add a bit of spice.

Anything that improves your well-being and increases your physical and mental stamina is yet another weapon in your defense structure. It is rarely "just one thing" that will improve or cure your pain, but a whole combination of factors that work together to achieve specific pre-set goals.

9. Finally, as a musician myself I was interested recently to read of a US study conducted by Lloyds Pharmacy which concluded that **music** can help relieve persistent, nagging pain for some people. The figures were especially high amongst 16 - 24 year olds who took part in the survey - a total of 66% - and the favourite type of music overall was pop, with songs such as Bridge Over Troubled Water by Simon and Garfunkel at the top of the leader board! Classical music came a close second, followed closely by rock and indie.

Listening to favourite songs can clearly help as a therapy, because it is embraces thoughts and feelings, memories and associations and as such has the power to be all-absorbing. On a physical level music expands the blood vessels, thereby improving blood flow and sending pain-relieving chemicals to the area of pain. Experiment to find out which particular music is your own personal "soul food", then make a point of incorporating it into your daily routine.

Sun Exposure

There is so much available information on the dangers of sun exposure and how to protect yourself against it that I doubt I can tell you much that you haven't heard before. However my main concern is the potentially harmful chemicals contained in "on the shelf" sunscreens used by the vast majority of people to protect their skin from UV rays. These chemicals can be very damaging to your skin, as their interaction with the sun's rays increases production of free radicals in your body *thereby potentially contributing to the development of those very skin cancers they are intended to protect against*.

So what are the alternatives, and how can you responsibly protect your skin without slathering on copious amounts of these toxic cocktails?

1. **Your front line of defense** is what you put into your body. All those foods that are high in anti-oxidants will offer you the best protection from inside, foods such as leafy green vegetables, colourful fruits, nuts and seeds and oily fish (see Section 1 chapter 5 on anti-oxidants to refresh your memory). Remember that tomatoes are better eaten cooked (especially in olive oil) or as a paste, sauce or soup. Cooking releases more of the anti-oxidant lycopene which they contain and which is so good for you.

2. **Take extra precautions** at the hottest time of day (usually from around 11.30 am through till about 2.00 – 3.00 pm). If you *are* outside at those times (which realistically, if you are on holiday, you probably will be) then cover up (even in water which does not automatically guarantee you immunity from the sun's rays) or stay in the shade.

Wear loose, cool clothing and **always** a hat. Darker coloured clothes with a tight weave absorb more UV rays than lighter ones so try to opt for these whenever you can. Invest in some fun and trendy cover-up items, complete with that ultimate finishing touch, the ubiquitous and enigmatic pair of shades.

3. Allow your skin **sensible access to the sun** at those times of day when UV rays are not at their strongest (usually early morning and late afternoon). This will allow your body to manufacture the vitamin D it needs for strong and healthy bones, and *to help protect you from the very same cancer that* **irresponsible** *sun exposure can cause*.

4. **Drink** plenty of fluids. You **must** remain hydrated, this is very, very important to remember. Still water is better than anything for this purpose. Keep a large bottle (preferably BPA free plastic, or a plastic alternative) with you at all times and replenish it frequently. I think it is widely accepted now, especially on the beach, that "cool people drink water". I cringe when I think of holidays in the past when a friend and I used to go to the beach for the day, armed with a couple of bottles of wine between us!

5. Remember that **cloud cover offers no protection from UV rays**, you can still burn through it, as you can also through water.

Similarly there is danger in snow, particularly if you are skiing in high altitudes. Here the sun's rays are largely unfiltered due to the poor quality of the atmosphere, so protection is very necessary.

6. **Certain drugs**, including some herbal remedies such as St John's Wort, can react with the sun against your skin. Always look up the side effects on the information leaflet provided with your medication, or check with your GP or with your pharmacist.

7. Use a **natural sunscreen** that contains all natural ingredients and no chemical blockers. Ingredients such as shea butter and jojoba oil, pure coconut oil, emu oil, sesame seed oil, green tea or aloe vera will all protect your body from free radical formation. Vitamin A too, can actually have a very positive effect on sun damaged skin, restoring surface levels in hours and it is the one ingredient in big brand-name cosmetics that I would actually give any credence to.

8. **Avoid sun beds**, and if you use a **self-tanner** then again opt for one that uses predominantly natural ingredients. Any product that reacts with your skin to actually change its colour must be pretty strong stuff and should be treated with suspicion! Remember, if it sounds too good to be true, it probably is!

9. As you become older, **be aware of any changes in your skin** in the way it reacts to sun exposure and do check your skin regularly for any unusual spots or moles that change shape or colour. If you notice anything out of the ordinary then **see your GP immediately**.

In conclusion to this section of the book I would say that: *you can either make a choice and make lifestyle changes, or you can prematurely suffer from debilitating and ageing diseases such as arthritis, heart disease or a stroke, which will all seriously impact on your looks, your skin and your whole demeanor as you become older.*

Of course if you are privileged to live to a ripe old age then this comes at a price sooner or later to many of us, but why make a down-payment? Read on for the final and arguably the most important piece of the jigsaw that will reveal a healthy and more youthful looking **you** …

Part Two: easy ways to incorporate these delicious foods into your diet that will stop - and even reverse - the signs of ageing

"All we are is the result of what we eat. Our diet is everything. What we eat is what we become ..."

As I said earlier, *our diet affects our whole body and as our skin is on show to everybody it is very visible evidence of poor nutrition and poor health.* As our diet, overall health and the condition of our skin are so closely linked, it probably comes as no surprise now to know that anti-oxidants (the lifeline of young, beautiful, and supple skin) also protect the body against cancer, a fact that at least half the people in this country have been found to be completely unaware.

By eating foods that are high in anti-oxidants you are therefore not only nourishing your skin but are protecting your body from illness and disease *"from the inside out".*

You may find it interesting at this point, to consider a race of people that not only age extremely well but have an incredibly long life expectancy -:

Look closely at any **Japanese** *person* and notice how smooth, even-textured and youthful their skin is. This flawless complexion is due to a combination of things, *a holistic approach to skincare* that has been practiced for centuries by oriental cultures in general and which is a lifestyle they have adopted to help them maintain beautiful skin.

This lifestyle is *aimed at prevention rather than cure,* and the major contributing factor is a *low fat but whole food diet* consisting mainly of fish (or other seafood) and vegetables such as bean sprouts, green peppers and sweet potatoes. These foods ensure *a major intake of anti-oxidants and zinc*, and the fish, apart from being rich in *omega 3 fatty acids*, supplies much needed moisture to the skin from its *healthy oils.*

The Japanese skin is also kept youthful with *protein* and *calcium* from tofu, soy products (made from fermented soy rather than processed) and yoghurt.

A further contributing factor is their consumption of *green and oolong teas* (up to 12 cups a day), *rich in both anti-oxidants and anti-inflammatory properties, and very protective to cell membranes.* While this may seem daunting to many western palates there are now numerous and varied preparations on our supermarket shelves. My own particular favorite is *green tea with blueberries from The Berry Company.* Drunk cold, this is very pleasant and refreshing, and leaves your mouth feeling much fresher than endless cups of "regular" tea and coffee. The Japanese consumption of coffee, alcohol and sugary drinks is minimal, and this very visibly reflects in their skin.

Think also, of **Mediterranean peoples**, with their love of fish, fruit, brightly coloured vegetables, salads, garlic, and olive oil - a plethora of foods from Nature's garden which keeps their skin supple and moisturized well into old age. Frozen or processed foods are hardly ever bought. Their fondness for rice, pasta and polenta keeps them fuller for longer, reducing the need to eat between meals, and like the Japanese they **drink a lot of water** to keep their skin hydrated and to flush out toxins.

It is interesting to note that a Mediterranean diet is often recommended as part of the rehabilitation period following a heart attack, as it is apparently even more effective in reducing cholesterol than to take a statin.

Motto: *It is not only what you put* **on** *your skin but what you put* **into** *it that matters.*

Regularly include the following foods in your diet to see a sensational improvement in the appearance and texture of your skin, and also your general energy levels and well-being. Whenever you can use fresh, organic food, in particular vegetables and fruit - but if this is not always possible then in the case of fruit and vegetables it is better to eat non-organic than not at all. Just remember that by doing so you risk exposing your system to toxins and chemicals from a multitude of pesticides. You may not be able to see them, but they are there and pose a very real threat.

The following lists are by no means exhaustive. Almost every type of fruit and vegetable contains a high proportion of one or more key vitamins, minerals or other nutrients supported by a complex balance of a myriad others that make each one such a nutritional powerhouse for your health and for your skin. I won't be going into every minute detail of what each single one contains, but want to make you aware of how potent these foods can be when eaten on a regular basis. Remember that good health equates to good skin, so anything that's beneficial to your health will also impact in a very positive way on the appearance and texture of your skin.

Fruits

The only downside to eating fruit, as with some vegetables such as carrots, is that most of its calorific content comes from natural sugars - so don't go completely OTT when including it in your diet, and if you are diabetic then you will of course recognize the need to be aware of those fruits that are particularly high in sugar, such as bananas.

Nevertheless, specific health issues aside, the nutritional benefits far outweigh a little indulgence and to substitute fresh fruit for processed sugary foods that have no nutritional value whatsoever is a hugely positive lifestyle choice to make. It is always best to eat fruit whole rather than juiced, in order to benefit from all the essential fibre it contains.

Home-made smoothies however, in moderation, make an easy, pleasant and nutritious drink so I have included them as yet another way in which you can incorporate some of the following delicious fruits into your diet.

- **apples**
- **apricots**
- **avocado**
- **bananas**
- **blackberries**

- **blackcurrants**
- **blueberries**
- **cantaloupe**
- **coconut**
- **goji berries**
- **grapefruit**
- **kiwi fruit**
- **papaya**
- **pineapple**
- **strawberries**
- **watermelon**

All of these delicious treats are jam packed with anti-oxidants and nutrients to nourish your skin and protect it from free radicals and cell (DNA) damage. Berries and kiwi fruits have probably the lowest sugar content of all. Buy them fresh (when in season) or, in the case of berries, frozen.

Apples are full of anti-oxidants such as vitamin C and beta-carotene, and are also detoxifying due to their anti-viral properties, hence the saying "an apple a day keeps the doctor away. Additionally they contain a rich and natural source of soluble fibre (most of which is to be found in the skin, so do not peel) and can help lower blood pressure and cholesterol. Like all crisp, crunchy fruit and vegetables they have a very beneficial effect on dental plaque.

- Enjoy anytime as a deliciously juicy snack (I love slicing apple and eating with small pieces of strong cheese) or add to fruit or green salads either sliced, chopped or grated.

○ There are also dozens of ways in which you can enjoy cooked apple, from a simple topping for hot or cold cereal or yoghurt, to home-made pies, crumbles, charlottes or cakes (made with unrefined ingredients of course!)

Apricots contain over 90% vitamin A, and some vitamin C in addition to calcium, potassium, copper and iron, the latter two of which help boost the levels of haemoglobin in your blood. Apricots also provide an additional source of *lycopene*, and their high fibre content helps to regulate the natural process of excretion.

○ Enjoy them lightly cooked in season, with a dollop of yoghurt or crème frâiche, or as a topping for hot or cold cereal.

○ Alternatively snack daily on a handful of organic, dried apricots, or dice and add to casseroles or other dishes for a Middle Eastern flavour.

○ Like many other fruits when in season, raw apricots can also be halved and added to green salads where they add not only flavour and texture, but colour for visual impact.

Note: dried apricots contain the same nutrients and natural sugar content (roughly 1 tsp in each apricot) as fresh.

Avocados are rich in mono-unsaturated fats (which are stored in your skin to protect its cells), a plethora of vital vitamins - especially vitamin E, the high content of which is largely responsible for the bright green colour of the fruits - and potassium, and as such they are a superb skin food that is one of your best weapons in your quest to keep your skin smooth and wrinkle-free.

They are low in sugar, high in fibre, and low down on the list of foods most affected by pesticides. As an added bonus they stimulate production of a substance called *glutathione* which blocks the absorption of bad fats.

- Halve and sprinkle with vinegar and a small amount of crushed sea-salt for a nutritious "anytime" snack, mash and spread as a topping on toast, or slice and add to salads.

- Avocado can also be used to make some delicious starters such as an avocado and prawn cocktail, plus it combines well with many fruits, in particular grapefruit. Use your inventive powers to the max!

Bananas are very useful as a source of instant, natural energy that lasts far longer than a quick chocolate fix. They do contain a large amount of natural sugar (about 7tsps in one banana) but are very rich in nutrients to counter-balance this.

They contain large amounts of soluble fibre to help bowel movements, and have a natural antacid effect in the body. They are a rich source of potassium and vitamin B6 (to regulate blood glucose levels and calm the nervous system) with moderate amounts of vitamin C *and polyphenolic anti-oxidant compounds* to help fight free radicals. They also contain iron, copper, magnesium and manganese, plus a protein called *tryptophan* that your body converts into *serotonin* to calm and relax your mood.

Bananas can be enjoyed anytime as a satisfying, healthy snack. While they are high in natural sugars and should therefore be eaten in moderation, when push comes to shove a banana carries far more health benefits than a bag of crisps or a piece of chocolate cake. In fact one banana has significantly more protein, carbohydrate, phosphate, iron, vitamin A and other nutrients than an apple! All of which enforces my point that you have to balance the negatives in certain foods against the positives when deciding whether or not to include them regularly in your diet.

- Banana makes a delicious addition to fruit salads, can be mashed as a topping for toast, sliced to make a tasty filling for pancakes, added to yoghurt, breakfast cereal or porridge (on its own or with other fruit such as blueberries) or even added to a curry ... the list goes on and on.

○ One of my favourite - and so easy treats is to slice a banana into a small dish of natural yoghurt, top with some crushed almonds and walnuts and sprinkle with a small pinch of cinnamon.

Blueberries are a rich source of vitamin C and *anthocyanins* which respectively repel pollutants and strengthen collagen. They rank as one of the top fruits and vegetables for anti-oxidant activity. The particular anti-oxidants in blueberries, also those in **blackberries** and **blackcurrants**, can apparently assist in fat reduction, and all berries are a source of soluble fibre which regulates both your digestion and blood sugar levels, and of potassium which can aid blood pressure control.

○ Fresh or frozen **blueberries** taste amazing when added to yoghurt and topped with a little granola or a few nuts, or stirred into porridge or other hot cereal.

○ Use whole or puréed blueberries as a topping for home-made or organic ice-cream, or to make smoothies.

○ And for a whole new taste sensation throw a few into a green salad and sprinkle over some crumbly cheese.

○ **Blackberries** are simply delicious when lightly cooked with apple, and enjoyed with hot or cold cereal, or yoghurt - and for those who crave a traditional pudding it is hard to beat a home-made blackberry and apple crumble.

○ **Blackcurrants** work well added to a large dish of mixed, stewed fruit sweetened with a little organic honey or agave nectar. Alternatively, they too can be puréed and added to hot or cold cereal or yoghurt.

Cantaloupe enjoys a massive 120% of vitamin A and 108% of vitamin C. It also contains niacin, vitamin B6 and folate, iron, calcium, potassium and essential dietary fibre. One of its key functions is to help with fluid retention by helping your body to excrete excess sodium, so a very useful fruit indeed!

○ Cut in half and remove the seeds, then spoon in some yoghurt or a scoop of organic ice-cream and sprinkle a small handful of raspberries or blueberries over the top.

○ Alternatively, cut the flesh into cubes and use in fresh fruit salads.

Coconut is currently bang on trend, being widely acclaimed by celebrities and dieticians alike as the latest "must-have" super food. It certainly ticks all the boxes for me as it is the perfect example of a real, whole food - an uninspiring looking little brown bomb of a fruit that practically explodes with *vitamins* (especially vitamin C and the B vitamins), *minerals* (potassium, magnesium and manganese, iron, copper, zinc, phosphate and selenium) and *electrolytes.*

It is very versatile as you can eat its "meat", drink its water and use its oil both in cooking and on your skin and hair.

Coconut Water is an excellent way to rehydrate your body after exercise, and Coconut Oil has both anti-viral and anti-bacterial properties embedded in its rich supply of *lauric acid.* Lauric acid is a (good) saturated fat that is known for its positive effects on the immune system when taken internally. Applied topically it will also ease skin conditions such as acne, eczema and psoriasis.

Most of the fat content of coconut oil is made up of MCFAs (Medium Chain Fatty Acids), which among their host of benefits for your health, work on your body's metabolism to improve thyroid function and assist a healthy weight loss. In addition coconut has the most delicious and naturally sweet taste, and can enhance the texture and flavour of many dishes.

- Before you can enjoy the wonderful benefits that coconut has to offer, you need to know how to (literally!) crack open the coconut. Firstly take a strong pair of scissors and using just one of the blades, prod the three little "eyes" at the end of the coconut. One will be less resistant and you will be able to gouge a small hole through which to extract the coconut water. That done, I find it easiest to double-wrap the coconut in a couple of plastic bags and smash it against a concrete surface such as steps, or a floor. This will usually break it into several pieces and allow you to prise the meat, or flesh, away from the shell with a strong knife. It can then be eaten plain as a snack, or grated and used in a wide variety of dishes such as soups, stir fries, porridge, yoghurt or breakfast cereal.

- Buy organic coconut milk for blending into curries or smoothies, and extra virgin coconut oil for cooking. There are actually a lot of quality coconut products around, so try your local health store or search online. Coconut water is also widely available on the supermarket shelves so if you don't fancy cracking open a fresh coconut, look out for the Vita Coconut brand which contains just natural coconut water.

Goji Berries, in spite of the fact that they are almost only ever to be found dried (this process normally takes place before export from parts of China, Mongolia and the Himalayas) are up there with most fresh fruits due to their very high anti-oxidant content, particularly that of beta-carotene. They actually taste much better than they look (they have the appearance of wizened little red berries) as they have a mildly tangy taste and a marvelously chewy texture that makes them perfect for snacking on at any time.

- If you like goji berries then try the juice, available at health food shops or at some Chinese herbal stores. You may also find the whole berries are available from these sources.

- Like most dried fruits you can also enjoy a handful sprinkled over cereal, porridge or yoghurt , or brew around a dozen or so in boiling water for 5-10 minutes (depending on preference) to make goji tea.

Grapefruit has been reported to help reduce insulin levels if eaten (or drunk, in the case of juice) before a meal. Pink Grapefruit in particular, is a good source of *lycopene*.

- Enjoy half a grapefruit lightly grilled with a drizzle of organic honey before breakfast or slice and add to salads where it blends particularly well with avocado.

Kiwi Fruit also contains anti-oxidants, including vitamin C, to support collagen and keep your skin smooth and firm. It also has low levels of natural sugar.

- Cut off the top like a boiled egg and scoop out the flesh for a really easy quick fix of vitamin C.

- Or slice and add to fresh fruit salads or smoothies.

- Always add Kiwi fruit to your fruit salad at the very last minute, as it contains enzymes that can cause other fruits to become mushy.

- Sliced Kiwi fruit also works very well in a green salad where it imparts a little natural sweetness.

Papaya also helps to renew collagen and elastin which gives your skin its springy texture, and is a source of the anti-ageing anti-oxidant *lycopene*.

- Arrange slices on a plate with half a lime and serve as a pre-breakfast treat. I first sampled this in Thailand, and have been eating it ever since. If you find papaya a bit messy to prepare, the dish works equally well with a lovely ripe mango.

- Alternatively use sliced papaya or mango in fruit salads and smoothies or as an exotic topping for some Greek yoghurt.

Pineapple is loaded with vitamins and minerals including vitamins A & C (both potent anti-oxidants), vitamins B1 & 6 (essential for the breakdown of sugars and starches in your digestive system, and for energy production), calcium, copper, phosphate, potassium and manganese. It is also rich in fibre, and *low* in fat, cholesterol, sodium and calories.

It contains *bromelain* which controls the level of acidity in digestive fluids and breaks down protein particles within food – thus keeping your digestive system nice and healthy. It is an amazing natural detoxifier, has strong anti-clotting and anti-inflammatory properties (I read recently that it is more effective against a cough than cough syrup) and is highly nourishing for your skin, hair, nails and teeth. It does however, have high sugar content so carries a caution for anyone who is diabetic or watching their weight.

- Pineapple is delicious eaten on its own, or as an ingredient in a mixed fruit salad (combine with some other tropical fruits such as mango and banana, and add a splash of rum for that tropical beach flavour!).

- Add to cottage cheese and eat as a light snack or an accompaniment to a green salad…or stir into natural yoghurt (on its own or in with other orange/yellow coloured fruits) for a quick and nutritious dessert.

- Pineapple also gives added zest to stir fries and curries, and is delicious lightly grilled to intensify its unique flavour.

Strawberries are rich in *ellagic acid* which helps to reverse the effects of pollutants in, for example, cigarette smoke, and can also help to prevent the formation of sun spots from UV. They are also a source of compounds known as *anthocyanins* which are responsible for giving the strawberries their red colour and which protect against UV rays and sun damaged skin.

- Add to fresh fruit salads, hot or cold cereal, or yoghurt - or simply enjoy on their own as a sweet and delicious snack.

- For a stylish yet effortless dessert, arrange some sliced strawberries in the centre of a plate, dust lightly with icing sugar to make them look pretty, and garnish with a sprig of mint – then around the edge add an artistic drizzle of the best balsamic vinegar you can afford, for decoration. If you haven't already tried it you may be surprised at how good it tastes. Most balsamic vinegars have a high level of sugar, so do shop around for one with the lowest sugar content you can find and use fairly sparingly. However balsamic vinegar does add a certain *"Je ne sais quoi"* to this simple and healthy dessert option.

Watermelon, a member of the same family as cantaloupe, pumpkins, squashes and cucumber, is another truly rich source of lycopene and anti-oxidants, particularly vitamin C. It is also a good source of magnesium and potassium and is renowned for its anti-inflammatory properties. You need to make sure you buy your watermelon when it is really ripe, as this increases the lycopene content. Watermelon has a "crunchy" deep pink flesh that, with a water content of over 90%, is refreshingly juicy and thirst quenching and makes a very significant contribution to your daily intake of fluid.

- The flesh of watermelon can be sliced, cubed or scooped into little balls with a useful little gadget called (not unsurprisingly) a melon-baller.

- It may be added to fruit or green salads, or combined with cantaloupe and kiwi for a refreshing chilled smoothie.

Vegetables

- **asparagus**
- **broad beans**
- **butternut squash**
- **carrots**
- **cauliflower**
- **celeriac**
- **courgettes**
- **fennel**
- **garlic**
- **greens**
- **leeks**
- **onions**
- **pumpkin**
- **sprouts**
- **sweet potato**
- **vegetable juices**

Asparagus is rich in vitamins A, C, E & K, vitamin B6, potassium, folic acid and chromium (necessary for the transportation of sugar into your body's cells). It is a tasty and extremely versatile vegetable.

- Use to make delicious winter soups, or add to wholegrain rice or pasta dishes.

- Asparagus also combines well with cheese and eggs to create starters or salads, and is a tasty accompaniment to any main meal when tossed with a knob of butter, a squeeze of lime juice and sprinkled with cracked black pepper.

- Make sure you do not over-cook this vegetable, the spears should still retain their shape when cooked. Limp, soggy asparagus is not the most attractive vegetable and will retain very few of its nutrients. Lightly steam rather than boil.

Broad Beans, surely one of the most delicious summer vegetables of all, have one of the highest levels of protein of any vegetable. They also contain a massive amount of dietary fibre to help maintain colonic health. They are a good source of vitamins A, C and K and offer a variety of minerals in the form of potassium, phosphorus, iron, magnesium and folate.

- Only cook broad beans until just fork tender, as over-cooking will deplete their nutritional content.

○ They can be boiled or steamed as a vegetable accompaniment to a meal in their own right, but also make excellent and tasty side dishes in combination with other foods such as asparagus, feta cheese and bacon with which they combine really well.

○ An easy and tasty summer dish is to mix broad beans with tiny new potatoes and toss in herb butter, or use ordinary butter and top with some fresh finely chopped thyme or parsley.

Butternut Squash is technically a fruit as it contains seeds. However as it is normally used as a vegetable I have included it in this section. It contains high levels of beta carotene, vitamin C and folic acid - with the seeds being a particularly good source of fibre - and is also a good source of mono-unsaturated fatty acids.

○ Squashes are a tasty and interesting accompaniment to meals, and can be roasted, puréed or baked in their skins with equal versatility.

○ They make particularly lovely soups where they combine well with other vegetables such as tomato, courgette, and sweet potato.

Carrots contain the highest beta carotene content (converted in your body to Vitamin A) and are also rich in anti-oxidants with an impressive supporting cast of essential minerals. They are a brilliant food for your skin, as they assist in the removal of toxins from the blood and effectively nourish and preserve the moisture content of, your skin's cells. Like most vegetables they are also high in fibre.

Carrots are actually better for you cooked than raw, as not only does the cooking process unleash up to three times more anti-oxidants than those in raw carrots, but the beta-carotene is significantly better absorbed.

- Steam rather than boil to preserve as many nutrients as possible.

- Carrots are extremely versatile and work well grated into salads or rice, sliced in stir fries or chopped in soups and casseroles.

- You can even add them to homemade cakes where they impart a natural sweetness, meaning you will need less sugar.

- And of course they provide a tasty accompaniment to any meal as a vegetable "on the side", whether boiled, steamed, braised, roasted or mashed, on their own or combined with other root vegetables. Carrot and parsnip mash is a delicious and nutritious alternative to regular mashed potato.

- Carrots are compatible with a wide variety of herbs and spices such as cinnamon, nutmeg, dill, tarragon or thyme. Try roasting with a few sprigs of thyme to bring out the natural sweetness of their flavour, or sizzle cooked and sliced carrots in a small pan with a knob of butter and a few cumin seeds for that extra bite.

○ You could also roast them glazed with a little butter and honey, or turn them into mash with a smidge of single cream and a sprinkle of nutmeg.

○ My own quick method of serving most steamed or lightly boiled vegetables for everyday meals is to drain and toss with a knob of butter, a squeeze of lime juice for extra vitamin C, and a sprinkle of ground black pepper - and carrots seem to respond particularly well to this treatment.

○ Orange too, brings out their wonderful sweet flavour … try cooking in a little fresh orange juice, maybe throwing in a few raisins for good measure dependent on the nature of the main dish. This is one vegetable where your imagination need know no bounds!

○ Buy organic carrots whenever you can, and don't scrape or peel as this action destroys many of the minerals that lie just beneath the surface of their skin.

Cauliflower is a highly nutritious vegetable which contains two unique nutrients: *indole-3-carbinole* and *sulforaphane.* These compounds work together to fight disease by flushing toxins from the body before they have a chance to develop into tumours. They are particularly effective in reducing the risk of prostate and breast cancers.

Like most vegetables cauliflower is rich in powerful anti-oxidants, namely vitamin C, beta-carotene and manganese. It also contains high levels of folate which is essential for healthy tissue growth and to maintain an efficient circulation, while vitamin K and omega 3 fatty acids work to decrease any inflammation both internally and at surface level.

Cauliflower also contains a cocktail of B group vitamins, and some supporting minerals in the form of phosphate and potassium. Insoluble dietary fibre helps to keep the digestive system in good working order, thus lessening the risk of constipation and other colonic diseases including cancer. *And it doesn't stop there …*

Glucosinolates and *thiocysanates* maintain the efficiency of the liver in the detoxification process, thereby helping it to zap potentially harmful substances before they become a problem, and *allicin* regulates the level of cholesterol in the body to reduce the risk of strokes and heart disease. Cauliflower is also anti-viral and anti-bacterial. Who would think that one vegetable could provide so many important benefits?

- Cauliflower, like most vegetables, is extremely versatile and can be boiled, steamed, baked or even fried.

- Use small florets in stir fries, as crudités for dips, or raw in salads with a little vinaigrette.

- Make a lovely thick winter soup with cauliflower and stilton … or of course the ever-popular cauliflower cheese (use equal parts cauliflower and broccoli for maximum anti-oxidant impact) can double as both a light lunch and a side-dish to a main course.

- My personal favourite is to shallow-fry small florets in a little olive oil and seasoning, stirring until golden brown and delicious! Add a squeeze of lemon juice if you like, or a little finely chopped garlic - in fact you could experiment by adding more or less any herb or spice that takes your fancy.

- Cauliflower is produced in large amounts in India, and the vegetable works particularly well with, for example, curry or cumin powder, maybe frying in coconut instead of olive oil.

- It may also be mashed in the same way as potato and this option is great for diabetics as it does not have the carbohydrate content of potato.

Celeriac or *Root Celery* is a member of the carrot family and closely related to the more common "leaf celery". It is very popular as a winter root vegetable with a distinctive yet subtle celery flavour, and although it can be a little daunting to look at with its rather grotesque and knobbly appearance it is actually very easy to prepare and cook.

Like most vegetables it is a very good source of fibre, and is also a particularly rich source of vitamin C, vitamin K and phosphorus plus some vitamin B6, magnesium and manganese, potassium, calcium and iron. It boasts many health benefits including protection from colonic cancer and immunity against the common cold, and it is also extremely important for the metabolism and maintenance of your body's cells (essential for good skin).

- The easiest way to prepare this vegetable is to wash/scrub gently to remove any surface soil, trim off the top and base then scrape off the outer skin with a sharp knife if preferred. You can then cut the entire root into quarters (as with potato, the free radical activity once the cut surface is exposed to air will turn the flesh brown, and this can be prevented by rubbing with a piece of lemon or immersing in cold water until cooking). The vegetable can now be sliced or chopped and added to many various dishes.

- Celeriac may be cooked and used as any other root vegetable. It is especially delicious boiled and mashed with a knob of butter, a pinch of unrefined sea salt and a twist of black pepper to make a tasty celeriac mash.

○ Alternatively mix with the same amount of mashed potato and serve with any meat or fish dish along with other root or green vegetables.

○ Celeriac may also be used in place of potatoes in soups or casseroles, and is tasty when added raw to salads, used to make coleslaw or grated as a garnish.

Fennel is a most interesting vegetable, a perennial herb plant that belongs to the parsley family (within the broader spectrum of herbs and spices) and can be used in a wide variety of cuisines, particularly well known in Italian and French dishes.

The bulb, used as a vegetable, has a rather crisp, crunchy texture and a slightly sweet and aniseed-like flavour. It is a good source of the anti-oxidant vitamins A & C, plus thiamine, riboflavin, pyridoxine and niacin. It also supplies calcium, iron, a host of other vital minerals and essential dietary fibre – and is valuable for its anti-oxidant and anti-inflammatory properties, all very good news for your skin!

○ This vegetable is simple to prepare, as all that is needed is to cut off the base (like an onion), remove the leafy stalks just above the bulb and then peel off the tough outer layers. The bulb can then be easily sliced, cubed or cut into strips before using in recipes such as soups, salads or stews.

○ Fennel can be thinly sliced to use either with dips or to add as "ribbons" to salads with, perhaps, avocado or in mouthwatering combination with orange and watercress.

○ Braised or steamed it adds a unique flavour to almost any dish, but is particularly delicious when teamed with salmon or other seafood.

○ Alternatively you could experiment with it as a side dish, for instance sautéed with some onions.

Garlic has so many health benefits that it's impossible to name them all within the context of this little book. Mainly, it is anti-bacterial, anti-viral, anti-fungal, anti-inflammatory and antiseptic, with properties that increase anti-oxidant activity in your body and fight free radicals.

Garlic also works to improve your immune function, and helps thin your blood to maintain a healthy heart and efficient circulation. **Note:** if you are on blood thinning medication and also eat a lot of garlic, you need to consult your GP or health practitioner as the two in conjunction could have adverse effects.

Garlic contains mega doses of vitamin C, vitamin B6 and manganese, also some iron, calcium, selenium, copper and a compound known as *allicin* which is responsible for much of the healing nature of garlic. It is an interesting fact that, although garlic has been comparatively slow to appeal to the British palate, extra garlic was grown throughout both the world wars, not to eat but to treat wounds.

The compounds of garlic responsible for its amazing health-giving properties are fully released upon crushing or chopping, so if you want to enjoy the full benefits of this wonderful little bulb then avoid cooking it whole. If you can, try to crush garlic about 15 minutes before eating, and if you are sautéing add the garlic near the end so you don't overcook it. Overcooking can virtually eradicate the potency of its nutrients. Raw garlic gives the most nutritional benefit, while the powdered and dehydrated versions contain very little.

- Garlic is widely used in a variety of ways to add its distinctive flavour to many meat, vegetable and seafood dishes, particularly those with a continental twist. Mediterranean countries use garlic as a staple ingredient in their cooking, adding it to soups, sauces, stews, risottos, pastas and stir-fries.

- Garlic is also use to create regional delicacies such as *aioli* (garlic mixed with egg yolks and olive oil), *ajoblanco* (garlic blended with almonds, oil and soaked bread) and a sauce common to eastern Mediterranean countries that is made of yoghurt with garlic and salt.

- Garlic can be added to various different types of bread, or to butter, to create delicious garlic bread, bruschetta and crostini.

- It works well with onions, tomato and ginger, especially in stir-fries and chutneys.

- Onion and garlic, sautéed gently together, are used as a base to which are added all the other ingredients for soups and casseroles so even if you don't like the taste of garlic, you should consider using it in this way where its flavour is not really very overpowering.

- Just remember that garlic cooks quicker than onions and will lose flavour if cooked for too long, so for best results add it near the end of the cooking time when the onions are almost soft.

Green Vegetables such as spinach, broccoli and kale are all excellent sources of vitamins A, B, C and E, calcium, potassium, iron, and magnesium to maintain the skin's PH for a beautiful, clear and luminous complexion. They are also full of fibre.

Note: if you are someone who drinks a lot of tea and coffee, then it is very important that you eat plenty of these dark, leafy greens in order to protect the absorption of iron in your body. Both tea and coffee contain natural plant compounds called *phenolics* which can hinder the uptake of iron, and ideally should be avoided for a couple of hours before or after a meal so as to minimize the risk of anaemia developing over the long-term.

○ Steam rather than boil for maximum nutritional benefit, and save the cooking water to add to soups or stews.

○ When cooked, toss with a knob of butter, a little lime or lemon juice (not just for flavour but for its vitamin C content which super-charges your uptake of iron from the leaves), and some black pepper. Or add a handful to casseroles, soups or salads.

○ *Savoy cabbage* makes a delicious side dish stirred through with some crème frâiche, grated gruyere cheese and a sprinkle of chopped nuts (pine nuts work very well with cabbage) or chopped and stir-fried with onions and lean, diced bacon.

○ Additionally *spinach* makes a very tasty filling for an omelette.

Note: when buying Kale and other strong leafy vegetables, make sure you look for young leaves, as the older ones can taste quite bitter.

Leeks belong to the alliaceae family alongside onions, garlic and shallots - although unlike their fellow companions they do not form bulbs. Although they have an onion-like taste, their flavour is altogether sweeter and more delicate so they are the perfect alternative for anyone who wants to enjoy the benefits of onions but with a milder and less pungent taste.

Leeks contain several anti-oxidant compounds that are converted into *allicin* via enzyme activity that occurs when the stalk is cut or crushed. Like onions and garlic therefore, they are anti-viral, anti bacterial and anti-fungal - not quite so potent, granted, but still a very significant anti-oxidant source.

Additionally leeks contain both soluble and insoluble fibre that works to keep your colon healthy and efficient. They are extremely high in folic acid, plus they contain several other B complex vitamins (in particular vitamin B6), vitamin A, and some smaller amounts of vitamins C, E and K. They are also a source of many vital minerals such as potassium, magnesium and manganese, calcium, iron, selenium and zinc. Most of these nutrients are to be found in the lower stem.

- Leeks are versatile vegetables that can be boiled, steamed, baked, stir-fried or roasted with equally delicious results. Depending on your tastes, boiled or steamed leeks have a softer texture coupled with a milder flavour, while sautéed or fried leeks are crunchier and firmer.

- *To sauté*, cut the leeks into equal pieces, then put a small amount of oil in a pan and heat until sizzling. Place the pieces of leek carefully into the hot oil and stir continually for around 15 minutes or until they begin to brown and feel tender when a fork is inserted. Remove carefully and add to soups, pasta, stir-fries, casseroles or any other savoury dishes of your choice.

○ For a different twist you could sauté a little fennel alongside, and serve as an accompaniment to a main course garnished with a squeeze of fresh lemon juice and some thyme.

○ Or, to make scrumptious buttered leeks, simply follow the method for sautéed leeks but using a couple of teaspoons of butter in place of oil, and adding a pinch of salt and some ground black pepper towards the end.

○ Leeks combine exceedingly well with most other vegetables, with sea-food, and with dairy products such as cheese, butter, cream and eggs.

○ They also make delicious soups such as leek and potato while sliced baby leeks or very young and tender stems can be added raw to a salad.

Onions, like garlic, have anti-oxidant, anti bacterial, anti-Inflammatory and laxative properties. They also help to maintain an efficient circulation. Also, like garlic, they are best eaten raw.

There are several different types of onions: red onions, white onions, green (spring) onions and yellow onions - and each type has a different vitamin/mineral content. If you are sufficiently interested or have specific health goals, then you should probably do some extra research on this, but suffice it to say that they are all jam packed with nutrients including a compound known as *quercetin* which is not only a powerful anti-oxidant flavanoid, but also has anti-inflammatory, anti-carcinogenic and anti-diabetic properties. It is found mainly in the outer layers of the onion, so do not over-peel.

- Onions are very versatile in that they can be eaten raw or cooked, boiled, fried, sautéed, baked, grilled, barbecued or pickled.

- They can provide an *accompaniment* to a meal - perhaps a zingy tomato and onion salad - a *vegetable side dish* of, for example, sliced and sautéed onions, the *key ingredient* in a meal such as french onion soup - or simply a *basic ingredient* within a recipe.

- You can use them in just about any savoury dish that you can think of. Chop, sauté and use in soups, casseroles, stir-fries and curries. Slice with plump, juicy tomatoes, mozzarella or feta cheese and some olives if liked, finished with a drizzle of olive oil, to create a mouthwatering Greek or Italian salad. The possibilities of this wonderful vegetable are endless.

Pumpkin (another vegetable that is technically a fruit!) contains high levels of vitamin E which make it a powerful anti-oxidant to reduce the effect of sun exposure and pollution on the skin. Vitamin A keeps your skin naturally moisturized and acts as a barrier against bacteria, and vitamin C promotes collagen production. The seeds themselves are rich in B vitamins, iron, phosphorus and zinc.

- o I recommend home-made pumpkin soup which is totally delicious.

- o You could also make a simple but hearty vegetable soup by roasting some chunks of pumpkin, carrot, parsnip and sweet potato in a little oil until brown, then transferring to a blender or liquidizer with some vegetable stock. Whiz until smooth and serve with a swirl of crème frâiche or soured cream.

- o Pumpkin flesh can also be puréed and used to make breads or cakes or to fill pasta, and it combines very well with butter, cream and other sweet fruits like apples.

- o It can, of course, be used as a vegetable accompaniment in its own right. Try frying it with some diced onion, diced pancetta and garlic for a tasty side dish.

253

○ Pumpkin seeds also, are really yummy and nutritious when lightly roasted in the oven. Alternatively buy good quality organic seeds from your local health store and eat as a snack or add to cereal, soups or casseroles.

Sprouts are one of the best sources of folic acid (needed for healthy blood) that you can find, and even if these are not your favourite vegetable the good news is that *just one sprout* will provide you with enough folic acid to last for 24 hours!

We have the Chinese to thank for the discovery of these vegetables many thousands of years ago, and they certainly help to keep you fit and healthy and strengthen your immune system. Apart from folic acid, they contain good amounts of anti-oxidants (notably vitamins A and C), a good range of B complex vitamins and high levels of vitamin K. They are a good source of vital health-giving minerals including iron, also some sulphur-containing compounds called glucosinolates that help combat cancer.

Sprouts are living foods and ideally should be picked fresh and stored straightaway in the refrigerator where they will continue to grow and actually increase their enzyme and vitamin content. If they are not refrigerated straight away then this process will reverse, which is why sprouts bought in the supermarket may have significantly less nutritional value due to being kept at room temperature for an unspecified length of time. In an attempt to rectify this, some unfortunate sprouts may even be treated with mould inhibitors so that they appear fresh to the consumer.

If you are unable - or have no desire - to try growing your own sprouts, then do try to buy them from sources like farm shops where they are likely to have been fairly recently picked, then refrigerate once you get them home.

○ Sprouts can be boiled, steamed, or roasted in a small amount of olive oil with a little salt. This latter method greatly intensifies their nutritional content, in particular that of vitamin K which becomes so potent that large amounts of fried sprouts can actually risk interfering with blood-thinning medications like Warfarin (consult your GP or a health specialist if you have any concerns).

○ However sprouts are, in my opinion, equally delicious boiled or steamed and combine especially well with the flavours of Christmas such as turkey, cranberry and nuts. Last year I bought some small pats of butter with orange and cranberry from M&S, and added one with a squeeze of lime juice to the cooked sprouts after draining.

○ Just be careful not to overcook as a sprout should hold its shape and form in the water. A soggy sprout is not a happy (or a nutritious) one!

Sweet Potato is classed as a vegetable rather than a starch, due to it's powerhouse of nutrients. It is packed full of anti-oxidants in the form of vitamins - especially vitamin A - and minerals. It is a good source of fibre which is needed by your body to promote an efficient digestive system, and it is also a low AGE carbohydrate. The beneficial effects of this will visibly reflect in your skin.

- Use sweet potatoes in place of regular potatoes as an accompaniment to meals. They work equally well boiled, steamed, baked or roasted brushed with a little olive oil and lemon juice, and are also very easily mashed.

- Make a cottage pie with lean mince or Quorn cooked with onions, garlic, peppers, courgettes and tomatoes, topped with sweet potato mash and grated, extra-mature cheddar cheese.

- Baked sweet potatoes too, are delicious hot or cold and work with both savoury and sweet toppings. The beta-carotene they contain is better absorbed with the addition of a little fat, so cheese-based toppings are ideal.

- For a sweeter alternative experiment by filling your baked potato with mashed banana in a little yoghurt topped with chopped nuts or a sprinkle of seeds, or try topping the banana with sprinkle of unrefined brown sugar and perhaps a hint of cinnamon or ginger, finishing off under the grill until the sugar caramelizes.

Vegetable Juices are simply full of anti-oxidant content and bursting with nutrients. They are also low in calories and make a tasty, nutritious and guilt-free drink that is lower in natural sugars than fruit juice.

○ Invest in the best blender you can afford (check out eBay or your local bargain pages for a good second hand model that doesn't cost the earth) and make your own vegetable smoothies to keep in the fridge – delicious power-drinks of a wide variety of veggies, nuts and seeds in a base such as coconut water or tomato juice. By blitzing whole vegetables you will also retain essential dietary fibre, so this is a great option for children or for anyone who has an aversion to eating a lot of vegetables. Always think, "if you can't eat it can you drink it?"!

○ If you don't want to make your own, then probably the best shop-bought version is *Vegesentials cucumber, pineapple & spinach smoothie* (from some branches of Waitrose) which, despite its rather murky green appearance, has a sweet and rather appealing taste. Although there are around 4tsps sugar contained in one bottle, this is not added sugar but stems directly from the natural ingredients. It also retains the pulp with its associated dietary fibre, so is a good occasional alternative. By all means look around for other juices when you are out and about, but beware of added extras such as salt.

Mushrooms

Mushrooms are in a category of their own as technically they are neither a fruit or a vegetable (they do not possess any of the necessary components of fruits or vegetables such as leaves, roots or seeds). Their method of reproduction is to release spores, and as such they are classified as belonging to the **fungus** family.

Apart from being a low calorie and low sodium food, mushrooms have important nutritional benefits, in particular for vegetarians as they are a rich source of protein. They are also high in essential fibre and contain a plethora of vitamins and minerals that do wonders for your overall health and for your skin. These include vital B vitamins including niacin (again, good news for vegetarians as certain B vitamins are not found in plant derived foods), vitamin D, phosphorus (which works with their high levels of protein), potassium, copper, zinc, magnesium and selenium. Mushrooms also contain *complex carbohydrates* that strengthen the immune system, and have known anti-inflammatory properties.

There are many different types of mushroom to tempt your palate, and each type has different levels of nutrients. I would recommend experimenting with a variety of different mushrooms for maximum nutritional benefits.

I would also strongly recommend that you buy organic, as mushrooms absorb any pollution from the ground in which they are grown. This means that if they were grown and harvested in a polluted area they will definitely contain toxins, and although these can be neutralized to a certain extent by the cooking process, there is no guarantee that it will remove them all. For this reason I would recommend that you always cook your mushrooms, not least because the cooking helps to process and release their various nutrients.

- My favourite way of eating mushrooms is to sauté them in a little olive oil or butter, a few minutes either side over a high heat until they are a nice golden brown and any liquid is reduced. You can add a bit of chopped garlic if you like and, right at the end of the cooking time, a little seasoning to taste.

- If you really want to push the boat out, then sauté with some chopped or sliced onions or shallots, or add a splash of sherry of a dash of red wine to the pan. Once they have been quickly cooked in this way the mushrooms can be added to almost any dish you fancy, for example, an omelette, scrambled eggs, soup, a topping for toast or a filling for a hot sandwich in place of or in addition to some meat.

○ Mushrooms are also wonderful roasted on a baking tray at about 450C for 15 to 20 minutes, and served as a side dish. The only preparation you need is to brush them lightly in oil (a tablespoon should be enough for around half a pound of mushrooms) and stir occasionally during the cooking time. Prepared this way, mushrooms are also delicious served on a bed of green salad, topped with grated parmesan, pine nuts and cracked black pepper. You can add your choice of either a light dressing, or a simple drizzle of balsamic vinegar.

○ Mushrooms may be sliced or chopped and added to stir fries, casseroles and risottos. If you are using a slow cooker for your casserole, add the mushrooms about half-way through to impart flavour and overall texture to the dish. Or, if you prefer to preserve the shape and form of the mushrooms, add them about half an hour from the end.

Salad Items

- **celery**
- **green and red "bell" peppers**
- **lettuce**

260

- **tomatoes**
- **watercress**

Celery is a leafy herbaceous plant frequently used in Mediterranean cuisines. It is simply bursting with good things including vitamins A, C and K, several of the B complex vitamins, folate, essential minerals, amino acids and fibre. It also contains some very specific anti-oxidants called *coumarins* which, together with vitamins A and C, provide a massive boost to your immune system. Part of the reason why so many people get coughs and colds during winter is because they don't eat enough fruit and vegetables to keep their immune system healthy.

The benefits of eating celery are many and varied. It has alkaline properties which means that it can maintain the PH of your body and counter any over-production of acid, and it also helps regulate your fluid balance. It is hydrating due to its high water content, and its glut of fibre keeps your gastro-intestinal tract primed and healthy and your cholesterol levels low. Its rich complex of B vitamins, supported by some of the vast array of minerals, promotes a restful night's sleep and helps to keep to your nervous system healthy.

In addition celery contains a specific chemical that works to decrease the level of stress hormones in your blood, keeping your blood vessels nicely expanded and your blood pressure low. All of these health benefits will, of course, reflect in the condition and vitality of your skin.

- The best time to eat celery is in summer when it is freshly in season and can be chopped and added to a summer salad or sliced and used as crudités for snacking on or for dipping.

- I love to fill the stalks with any soft cheese sprinkled with a little paprika, which makes a delightful snack or appetizer. Peanut butter also works well for this purpose.

- Short sticks of celery offered with a cheese board after a meal make a refreshing change from grapes, and are actually better for you. Not only does celery refresh the palate but it also helps to reduce the build up of plaque on tooth enamel. I simply serve it in a small glass of water on the side to keep it crisp and appetizing.

- Celery is also delicious when chopped and used to add texture to sandwich or baked potato fillings such as tuna or chicken with a little mayonnaise. One of my favourites is chopped celery added to a mixture of grated cheese, grated apple and bound with a smidge of mayonnaise. You can also add a sprinkling of nuts such as walnuts, or a few dried raisons if you wish, for some extra nutrition.

- Celery adds a delicious crunch to vegetable stir fries, combined with, for example, carrots and onions, small florets of cauliflower and broccoli, thin slivers of bell peppers, chopped chilli peppers, garlic, ginger - the possibilities are many and varied.

○ Serve as a side dish, or combine with a little low sodium soy sauce and serve with brown rice, wholewheat pasta or tofu as a main course.

○ Celery can also be chopped and added to soups or casseroles. In order to preserve the optimum nutritional value, as with most vegetables it is best to chop just before use rather than to prepare ahead and store in the fridge. Steaming preserves far more vitamin and mineral content (as much as 99% after 10mns) than submersing in boiling water.

○ Finally, for a refreshing, hydrating drink that will not only replace those essential minerals and salts, for example after strenuous exercise, but will help control the need for sweet, sugary foods, drink a glass of freshly squeezed celery juice – it gives your mouth a real "zing"!

Green and Red "Bell" Peppers (technically fruits as they contain seeds) offer large amounts of beta-carotene and vitamin C, also some vitamin E, vitamin K, B vitamins and essential minerals. Red peppers contain a much higher proportion of nutrients - in particular beta-carotene - than green peppers and are also a good source of the anti-oxidant *lycopene*.

263

- Raw peppers add fresh, crunchy texture to any salad, and make ideal crudités to snack on or use as tasty dippers.

- They can also be added chopped or sliced to sauces, casseroles and stir fries during the cooking, or roasted and used to make delicious Mediterranean style soups.

- Red peppers in particular, are delicious roasted with a little olive oil, seasoning and a sprinkle of thyme, then added chopped to scrambled eggs or omelettes … or combine with a soft cheese for a delicious and nutritious sandwich filling.

- Peppers are also good grilled with a light brushing of oil and a little unrefined sea salt, or season and add splashes of colour to grilled or barbecued kebabs.

- And of course stuffed peppers are a tasty meal in themselves, filled with, for example, some crumbled feta cheese, chopped black olives and tomatoes, drizzled with olive oil then roasted in the oven until tender and melting.

Lettuce is very underrated by many people who assume that it contains nothing but water. Well even if this were true, its 95% water content alone is very good for you and counts as part of your daily fluid intake.

However lettuce is a very important source of anti-oxidants, vitamins and minerals - in particular beta-carotene and folate – with **Rocket** having probably the highest vitamin A content in addition to being rich in vitamin C and potassium. **Romaine** is also high up there at the top of the leader board for anti-oxidant content. Because lettuce is eaten in its raw state we reap the full benefits of all it has to offer. Tear and shred by hand rather than cut the leaves, as this releases a higher proportion of nutrients.

○ Experiment with different types of lettuce as they all have different textures and taste – even varying shades of green. As a rule of thumb those lettuces with the darkest leaves are the best sources of beta-carotene.

○ Use a variety of leaves in a simple green salad accompanied with good quality olive oil (to aid the absorption of vitamin A), balsamic vinegar and a small sprinkle of salt …

○ … or shred a whole lettuce and add to soups such as spinach, leek or avocado.

○ Buy organic whenever possible, as lettuce (a favourite food of slugs!) is high on the list of foods containing pesticides.

Tomatoes, like peppers, are also technically fruits. They are one of the best sources of the anti-oxidant *lycopene*, especially when eaten cooked or in a paste.

They also contain vitamin C, vitamin E, beta-carotene and potassium.

- Use as a basic ingredient in soups, stews and pasta dishes, also add slices of tomato to the top of almost any dish before cooking. This works particularly well with dishes such as home-made moussaka, lasagna, cauliflower cheese or any dish topped with mashed potato or grated cheese.

- Always think, "can I add tomato to this dish before cooking?" If you do this, then you will be adding some valuable anti-oxidant activity!

Watercress is, in my opinion, a super food among super foods. It boasts a densely concentrated nutritional package that contains high levels of vitamins A, C, E and K plus calcium, potassium, manganese, magnesium and phosphate. It is also an exceptionally rich source of iron.

In addition watercress contains the disease-fighting *phytochemicals* that are present in other leafy vegetables such as broccoli and cabbage, and as a natural antibiotic can help smooth out any blemishes and diminish the appearance of pores on your skin. It is great for use as a detox, and best eaten raw to lock in the maximum nutritional benefits.

- Use raw in green salads with a dressing of your choice (something like sweet lime really complements the unique peppery flavour of the watercress), or combine with fresh fruits like satsuma or pear, or with grilled goat's cheese, to make an unusual and tasty starter.

○ Watercress also packs a crunchy punch when chopped and added to whole-meal sandwiches. It combines well with fillings such as salmon, tuna or soft cream cheese with chives.

○ You can also use it to make delicious soups, either on its own or blended with peas, asparagus or potato - or add to melon or pear smoothies, to omelettes where it adds flavour and texture, or to fillings in baked potatoes.

Finally, while I'm sure you all know how to make a salad you might like to copy my mega version which includes a plethora of both traditional salad items and fresh fruits "prepared on the plate":

○ In summer in particular I like to make this large mixed salad of lettuce, sliced or chopped cucumber, celery, tomato, watercress, peppers, and whatever else I have in at the time.

○ Depending on my choice of protein (lean white meat, salmon, eggs or cheese), and also on the time of year, I might then add a small amount of any (or all!) of the following: chopped or sliced apple, organic grapes, kiwi fruit (blends particularly well with salad), avocado, strawberries, fresh or dried apricots, grapefruit and yes, even chopped banana!

○ Sprinkle over some chopped nuts or a few seeds, add a squeeze of lime juice and some freshly ground black pepper.

And there you have it, a delicious, easily prepared and low calorie meal that is not only interesting to look at and to eat but is absolutely jam-packed with nutrients for your skin.

Tip: *As there will be a lot of ingredients, have them all to hand before preparing.*

Seafood

- **salmon**
- **shellfish**
- **tuna**

Salmon is truly a super food, a key source of o*mega 3 and fatty acids* that keep your skin supple. Unlike canned tuna, canned salmon retains most of its omega 3 content. Fatty acids form part of the epidermis where they help maintain a firm, water-proof surface that locks in moisture. They are therefore essential to preserving the moisture content and integrity of your skin as you get older, and in addition can help to lower your heart rate and blood pressure.

Salmon also contains essential nutrients for plumped up healthy skin including EPA (*eicosapentaenoic acid*) which the body converts into prostoglandins to prevent inflammation, *selenium* to protect from sun exposure, and *protein* for the production of collagen. There are so many ways to enjoy this delicious food so try to eat at least three to four servings a week.

Mackerel, trout, sardines and herrings are also good sources of omega 3. If you are vegetarian or don't like fish, then the best nutritional alternative is tofu which is rich in calcium and iron and contains virtually no sodium or saturated fat.

I do have some reservations about tofu for the same reasons as soy beans, but vegetarians have a comparatively limited choice of staple foods compared to meat-eaters as it is, which is why it is not on my "hit list"! Do, however, try to choose quorn products in preference when you can.

- o Lightly steam, grill, poach or oven-cook oily fish, remembering that a lower heat will preserve its omega 3 fat content. Salmon in particular, tastes wonderful cooked for around half an hour in foil with lemon juice, a smidge of olive oil and some herbs such as dill or parsley - or pan fried with freshly squeezed lemon or lime and served with watercress or other green leaf salad.

- o Salmon can also be teamed with a home made parsley, dill or watercress sauce and some fresh vegetables such as asparagus, broccoli or green beans (steamed or stir-fried) for a healthy and delicious meal.

○ If you prefer a sweeter more exotic taste, coat it in a little organic honey and soy sauce before cooking and serve with crisp, stir fried vegetables.

○ Or for a quick and tasty snack, mash cooked salmon with a smidge of olive oil, some lemon or lime juice and some seasoning to taste, then spread on toast (this also works well with mackerel and sardines).

○ If you do not eat fish then as mentioned above, tofu is a very versatile and nutritious alternative. Firm tofu is good for stir frying or adding to soups and sauces, while the softer ones are good for mashing, chopping & adding to salads.

Shellfish, for instance prawns, scallops or crab, are a wonderfully rich source of minerals, especially zinc which is vital to help your skin's renewal and repair, and to regulate its oil production. They are also rich in selenium. It is worth noting that the most sustainable shellfish are mussels, oysters and crab, and when buying prawns then look for king or tiger prawns that are organically certified.

○ Shellfish can be rather intimidating to prepare and cook as they seem to be quite fiddly or even messy, however a prawn cocktail is not that difficult to make as a starter and it is easy to add just a few prawns to a salad or sandwich for a quick mineral fix (they combine very well with avocado).

o   When eating out, mussels in white wine and garlic is one of the tastiest dishes I know for seafood lovers, and scallops are to be found on most menus nowadays, although unless you know their source they are very likely to have added water and chemical*s*.

Tuna is an excellent source of protein and omega 3 fatty acids, both excellent skin foods. It also contains vitamins B6, B12 and niacin, vitamin K, phosphorus and potassium. Note however, that it is naturally quite high in sodium so if you are particularly fond of tuna then try to vary your lunchtime sandwiches from time to time!

Canned tuna unfortunately, has greatly reduced levels of omega 3 which is affected by high temperatures used in the canning process, so if you are eating tuna for its omega 3 content then you need to opt for the fresh variety. However canned tuna still contains high levels of protein and is much better for you than red meat.

o   Like salmon there are so many ways to enjoy this delicious and versatile food. It makes wonderfully tasty sandwiches when drained and mashed with a small amount of mayonnaise (pick one with the lowest fat/sugar/salt content that you can), and some ground black pepper.

- ○ It is also a popular addition to salads, bound with mayonnaise and combining with, for example, chopped celery and white beans - or simply dress with a little lemon juice or malt vinegar.

- ○ Of course the classic tuna salad is the Salad Niçoise, made of chunks of freshly cooked tuna with hard boiled eggs, potatoes and crunchy green beans on a bed of lettuce, onion and tomato – delicious!

- ○ Fresh tuna is also nutritious and tasty when lightly grilled and served with a green salad and baby potatoes, or try the recipe in the bonus section at the end to enjoy it rather more unusually with a serving of hot fruit.

Dairy Produce

- **cheese**
- **eggs**
- **milk**
- **yoghurt**

Cheese, even though it is given bad press for its cholesterol, sodium and saturated fat content, is actually a whole and natural food and a very important source of nutrition. *It cannot be compared to "junk" foods like crisps or chips which are laden with "baddies" yet have little nutritional value.*

Cheese is a recognized high source of phosphorus and protein, the two of which work together to develop and maintain healthy cell structure throughout your body. It also contains vital amino acids, some of which cannot be found in plant foods, and is a rich source of calcium with particularly high levels present in hard cheeses. It supplies your body with vitamins A, D, E, K and several of the B complex vitamins, notably vitamin B2, B6 and B12.

The concentration of vitamins does depend on the fat content of the cheese, with most low fat varieties (as you would expect) offering a significantly lower proportion of nutrients and high quality protein. **Partially skimmed mozzarella** is an exception as, although lower in fat and calories, it actually has a very similar protein content to full fat cheese.

If you are watching your sodium intake then avoid in particular, blue cheeses and parmesan which carry particularly high amounts. **Goat's cheese, cheddar** and **mozzarella** are some of the best choices as having less than 200mg of sodium per ounce.

If you are lactose intolerant, then it is not all bad news as ripened cheese like Cheddar naturally contains only around 5% of the lactose found in whole milk, while aged cheeses contain almost no lactose at all. As always if you have a medical condition, check with your GP or dietician before making any changes in your diet.

- ○ I'm sure I don't need to tell anyone how to enjoy cheese as it is one of the world's favourite and most widely indulged foods. However do eat it sensibly and as part of a healthy, balanced diet - and if you are one of those people who can't leave it alone when it is in the fridge, then avoid pre-packed cheese and buy only a very small amount at a time from the deli counter.

- ○ As mentioned before, cheese is very good at neutralizing the acids that cause dental plaque, so a small piece after dinner, especially with an apple, or piece of carrot or celery, is a good way to end your meal.

Eggs (not strictly dairy I know, but included here for ease) are also packed with protein - especially the whites - while the yolks are rich in vitamin A. This is a fat-soluble vitamin that will be better absorbed by your body when eaten alongside some healthy fats such as avocado. Eggs are also rich in selenium and zinc, and are one of the few dietary sources of vitamin D.

- ○ Eggs can be boiled, poached, fried, baked or scrambled.

- ○ They may be enjoyed on their own with whole-grain buttered toast for breakfast, made into omelettes or frittatas, or used in a whole spectrum of sauces, custards and baked goods.

○ A very simple starter dish is to boil, grill or steam some asparagus spears and top with a poached egg before sprinkling over a little lemon juice and black pepper.

Please do not support the battery/caged hen industry – buy organic, free range eggs which are so much nicer and better for you, and can be purchased almost everywhere for very little more than the cost of battery eggs.

Milk too, is a good source of vitamin A, and also contains protein, essential for building new cells. *Buy organic* to increase the amount of polyunsaturated fatty acids.

○ Add to cereal, porridge, soups and smoothies or puddings, or simply drink a small glassful once or twice a day.

Yoghurt maintains a healthy digestive system that will work efficiently to flush out toxins from your body. Free of "sludge", your skin will be helped to regain its elasticity and become smooth and wrinkle free. Yoghurt is also another good source of zinc, and vitamin A to promote healthy skin.

○ Enjoy with almost any kind of raw or cooked fruit for a delicious and nutritious "anytime" snack. Chopped banana is particularly beneficial as banana is a source of inulin, a carbohydrate that enhances the probiotic action of natural yoghurt.

○ Alternatively use swirled into soups or stews, to make dips or sauces or even stirred into porridge.

Nuts and Seeds

- **almonds**
- **brazil nuts**
- **cashew nuts**
- **hazelnuts**
- **peanuts**
- **pecans**
- **pistachios**
- **walnuts**

Nuts and Seeds are excellent sources of omega 3 Fatty acids. Although high in fat, most of the fat they contain is of the mono-unsaturated variety which promotes good health, and their powerhouse of nutrition means that to omit them from your diet due to the common misapprehension that they are bad for you, is to deprive your body of some of its most potent nutritional sources.

Almonds are high in calcium, vitamin E and riboflavin, particularly important for the skin. They are also **gluten free**.

- Add a handful of whole almonds to stir-fries, porridge or couscous or for a delicious and healthy snack, melt some good quality dark chocolate and use to coat some wedges of apple, then roll in crushed almonds.

Brazil nuts have exceptionally high levels of selenium and unsaturated fatty acids, which protect your skin from free radical damage caused by sun and pollution and significantly reduce inflammation. Even just one or two a day will give you the recommended daily allowance and provide benefits that experts think may last for up to 30 days.

- Coarsely grind or chop, depending on intended use, and add to soups, salads, cereal or porridge, fruit cake mix or crumble toppings.

- Or simply eat a few every day as a delicious snack.

Cashews are rich in iron, zinc, copper and magnesium, and have high levels of monounsaturated fats. They are therefore excellent in promoting anti-oxidant activity and energy production, plus they help keep your blood pressure low and your heart healthy. All this of course, encourages good circulation which is vital to maintaining the condition and smooth functioning of your skin.

- Cashew nuts can easily be broken into small pieces and added to salads or stir-fries, lending themselves well to oriental dishes such as Thai or Chinese.

○ Try stir-frying and adding to whole grain rice, or making a paste by soaking in water (enough to cover), then mashing and stirring into curries or casserole dishes.

○ Like most nuts cashews taste wonderful when roasted on a baking tray in the oven for five to ten minutes at around 350 - 450 degrees, and no extra oil is needed!

○ Because they have a rather richly luxurious and succulent flavour, they also work very well in puddings, and I sometimes scatter some over the top of a trifle or add to a crumble mix.

Hazelnuts are also known as **filberts** or **cob nuts**. They have a deliciously sweet, nutty flavour and are simply packed with nutrients, in particular vitamin A, vitamin E and exceptionally high levels of folate. They also contain many vital minerals including copper, manganese and iron - and are of course, a rich source of essential dietary fibre. Like almonds they are g**luten free**.

Hazelnuts are best bought unshelled rather than processed and pre-packed, as potentially harmful chemicals are often used in the processing procedure. Unshelled they will store for years in a cool dry place. If you do buy them ready shelled however, keep in an airtight container in the fridge to prevent them going rancid due to the amount of oil they contain. This oil, often used in cooking where it imparts a wonderfully nutty aroma to the food, is commonly used as a base oil which works to protect and hydrate the skin.

○ Hazelnuts can be eaten on their own (or roasted and salted) as a nutritious snack, or chopped and added to cereal, porridge or crumble toppings.

Peanuts are bursting with protein and anti-oxidants, but eat the unsalted variety or you will cancel out most of their health benefits. They are richer in anti-oxidants (including the powerful anti-oxidant *reservatrol* found in red grapes or red wine) than many fruits, and this anti-oxidant activity can be made more potent still by roasting.

More than three parts of the fat contained in peanuts is the healthy monounsaturated variety such as *oleic oil* found naturally in olive oil. They are also a good source of fibre, vitamin E, niacin, folate and manganese.

○ The easiest way to incorporate peanuts into your diet is a handful every day as a snack, but they are also delicious chopped and sprinkled over salads and into stir fries.

○ Peanut butter in moderation, is a tasty topping for toast or as a filling in celery sticks. Buy this organic - it should contain nothing but peanuts and salt – and make it last. You should not over-indulge due to the high sodium content, and if you are on a low sodium diet then seek advice from your GP or a Dietician.

○ Avoid any low fat varieties as they will contain added sugar. One of my favourite brands is Whole Earth Organic which contains all natural ingredients (peanuts, palm oil and sea salt) and no added sugar.

Pecans are one of the best nuts of all for providing anti-oxidant benefits, as they contain a high level of *phyto-chemical substances* that serve to enhance your body's general anti-oxidant activity. They also contain vitamin A, vitamin E and many of the B complex vitamins, plus a wide range of essential minerals and dietary fibre. Over 90% of the fat they contain is of the healthy mono-unsaturated variety, and they have an amazing zero level of sodium and cholesterol.

○ Pecans have a lovely luxuriant and buttery taste and are delicious eaten as an everyday snack or used in any of the ways suggested above.

Pistachios, as with all nuts, offer excellent levels of protein, fibre, vitamins and minerals. They offer substantial amounts of mono-unsaturated fatty acids in addition to many of the B complex vitamins, vitamin E, carotenes and complex polyphenolic anti-oxidant compounds. They are also a powerhouse of minerals, with particularly high levels of iron and copper.

- ○ Buy pistachio nuts semi-open, or you'll need to use a nutcracker!

- ○ Pistachios are great to snack on - quite addictive, in fact - or added to fruit or vegetable salads.

- ○ They are also delicious roasted and crushed, and sprinkled over desserts or into crumble toppings, cake mixes etc.

Walnuts add their unique flavour and crunch factor to many foods. Like most nuts they are an excellent source of mono-unsaturated fatty acids such as *linoleic acid*, which assists in keeping your skin water-tight and increases the amount of good cholesterol in your body to help keep your blood pressure nice and low. They also contain vitamin E, vitamin B6, magnesium, calcium, iron and zinc.

Eaten regularly they support your immune system and are also thought to contain anti-cancer agents, while their anti-inflammatory properties are particularly beneficial to skin diseases like eczema and psoriasis.

To remove the shells at factory level often involves a chemical process that should be avoided if at all possible. Rather than purchasing bags of ready-shelled nuts therefore, it is better to opt for loose, unshelled nuts and invest in a good old-fashioned nutcracker!

- ○ Walnuts can be enjoyed simply as a snack, and like all nuts a handful a day provides a potent shot of all their health giving nutrients.

- ○ They pack a powerful punch when lightly toasted, chopped and added to salads, pasta, breakfast cereal or porridge, and they add crunch to yoghurt or any fruit-based dessert.

- ○ Walnuts also combine extremely well with mushrooms in, for example, a stroganoff.

Basically, if you are by now suffering from information overload with regard to nuts, just remember this: if you make or consume any of the following – salads, stir fries, pasta, bread, cakes, pancakes, cereal, yoghurt, ice cream, soft cheese, fruit salad, crumbles, soups, casseroles or vegetable dishes, then just add a handful or sprinkling of nuts (whole or chopped depending on the dish) to add a powerful shot of nutrition and anti-oxidant content. with no extra effort.

Seeds - an overview

All seeds are highly nutritious and power-packed with a rich concentration of vitamins, minerals and dietary fibre.

One of my favourites is *fennel seeds* which have that lovely sweet and fruity aroma when rubbed gently between the fingers. They are often used in India as part of curry powders, but may be lightly roasted or ground and added to flavour many different sorts of recipes. They also impart a uniquely different taste to breads and cakes (added to the dough or cake mix before cooking), or to savoury biscuits and cheese.

Note: the compounds in fennel seeds may be neuro-toxic in large quantities, and pregnant women may be advised not to eat too many due to the concentration of oestrogenic compounds they contain. However unless you eat massive amounts of fennel you are unlikely to come to any harm and, as always, if you are pregnant or have an underlying medical problem then do check with a health specialist if you have any concerns.

- o **All** seeds can be eaten as snacks or easily incorporated into your daily diet by adding to many dishes including soups, salads, stir fries, casseroles, desserts, porridge or breakfast cereal.

- o Browse your local health shop and experiment to find those you like the most, then use regularly to notice a real difference in your skin.

- o As with nuts, just think "what can I add them to?" A small sprinkle to either savoury or sweet dishes is all that is needed to reap the amazing benefits of these wonderful foods of nature.

○ Incidentally don't forget **black cumin seeds** which, as mentioned earlier, have strong anti-inflammatory properties and can make a significant difference if added regularly to your diet.

Lean White Meat

- **chicken**
- **turkey**

Chicken, when responsibly reared, is a very important source of protein, both with or without its skin, and being a low AGE food is a very healthy choice unless of course, you deep fry it in large amounts of oil. It also contains vitamin B6, niacin and selenium plus some calcium, potassium and phosphorus, and it is low in sodium. Its only downside is that it is naturally *high in cholestero*l, however as with any food, unless you have an underlying medical problem and as long as you eat sensible amounts, this should not need to be an issue.

As discussed earlier, in order to be sure that you are buying quality chicken you need to look not only for organic but also pasture-raised birds, and preferably locally sourced. They have a massively higher nutritional content.

○ Chicken is very versatile and may be baked, grilled or roasted, before adding (hot or cold, sliced, cubed or in portions) to salads, roasts, barbeques, soups, sandwiches, stir-fries or kebabs.

○ If roasting, try rubbing the chicken all over beforehand with lots of fresh lemon juice and a little unrefined sea salt.

Turkey is choc-a-block with all manner of goodies for your health and your skin. Apart from being low in saturated fat it is a great source of protein, and contains significant amounts of riboflavin, niacin and vitamin B6, zinc, selenium and phosphorus. It plays an important role in boosting the immune system, and as with chicken its only downside is that it is naturally *high in cholesterol*. Unlike chicken however, it is also *high in sodium*, so if you have to watch your sodium intake for medical reasons then chicken would be the better option.

○ Use pretty much as for chicken.

○ A neat way to use left-over turkey is to combine it with slices of fresh mango, a green salad and some cashew nuts (oven roasted for around ten minutes at 180c/Gas Mark 6) – an interesting alternative to the ubiquitous turkey casserole!

Whole-wheat Foods

Whole-wheat foods are those made from flour that still contains the kernel, or "germ", that is found within the wheat grain. This is normally destroyed during the manufacturing process, which appears senseless as it is the part of the grain where the majority of nutrients are to be found.

Wheatgerm contains a powerhouse of vitamins and minerals, including vitamin E, vitamin B6, thiamine, folate, magnesium and manganese, copper, phosphorus, potassium, zinc and an impressive amount of iron. It also provides dietary fibre and protein, and is one of the best sources of omega 3 fatty acids that you can find.

- I cannot stress enough, the benefits of taking wheatgerm as a supplement. You can blend it into regular flour or breadcrumbs, smoothies, pancake mix, crumbles, soups or casseroles or simply sprinkle it on breakfast cereal or in yoghurts.

- **Always choose organic wholewheat bread and pasta** which are both far healthier and more nutritious than their wishy washy counterparts.

Obviously if you are intolerant to wheat or worried about its AGE inducing properties, then you will have to choose some wheat free alternatives and make up the nutritional value from other foods.

Oats

Oats provide essential soluble fibre that can help lower any "bad" cholesterol levels, and they are known to de-stress the skin and greatly enhance its complexion. Wholegrain oats in particular, also reduce the build-up of plaque on the walls of your blood vessels and have been proven to significantly lower blood pressure.

- Eat as porridge or add a heaped tablespoon to plain yoghurt, smoothies, cereals or the topping for fruit and savoury crumbles.

- Use oats in place of breadcrumbs in recipes, and add to thicken soups and casserole dishes.

Raw Foods

Raw foods have been hailed in the past as your skin's best kept secret, and to a large extent this is indeed true. Do you remember we talked about the skin being a mirror of your overall health and wellbeing? Well, a cheap and so easy way to see a rapid improvement in your skin's texture and luminosity is to eat raw fruits and vegetables - they have a high natural moisture content which is a really cool way to moisturize your skin from the inside.

However this issue can sometimes be rather confusing, as while cooking food can damage some of its essential compounds it can also help in the release and absorption of others, namely anti-oxidants such as lycopene. This is particularly true of carrots, mushrooms and spinach. Carrots and spinach both lose vitamin C content during cooking, but enjoy a boost of vitamin A and lycopene.

Onions and garlic on the other hand, are certainly better eaten raw - as is broccoli which contains an anti-cancer enzyme that is damaged by heat – while a cupful of raw, shredded cabbage just once a week is sufficient to protect you against colon cancer.

- My own solution to this little dilemma is to lightly cook my vegetables in the normal way, but also to eat them raw as "nibbles" (for instance while preparing the vegetables to cook for dinner!) and in salads – thus getting the best of both worlds! If you can do this you will look better, feel better and have so much more energy.

Green and Herbal Teas

Green or herbal teas contain important anti-oxidants. Green tea in particular contains an anti-oxidant called *catechin,* also p*lant polyphenols* which boost circulation to your skin.

Just a word of caution for anyone who takes medication for blood pressure or hay-fever, as it has been discovered that the plant chemicals in the drink can interfere with the absorption of certain of these medications. If this applies to you I would advise that you ask your GP before starting to drink this tea in any great quantities.

- Add some fresh natural fruit juice to green tea and chill for a refreshing, nutritious drink.

Still Water

Still water is so important to the health and appearance of your skin that I cannot emphasize it enough. "Hydration, hydration, hydration" is the key to a smooth, radiant and supple skin that will defy the ageing process and stop it in its tracks. Aim to drink two litres a day. I almost always now drink bottled water, although if in a plastic bottle I decant the contents into a BPA free container.

- If you find it difficult to drink a lot of water, rather than drink a whole glassful at a time you might find it easier to use a straw and sip small amounts throughout the day.

- You could also drink ***coconut water*** which (as previously mentioned) is an excellent way to rehydrate your body, particularly after exercise. Pure coconut water is absorbed very easily by your body as it is *isotonic* and *sterile*, and therefore very similar to blood plasma (it has been used intravenously in emergency situations for over 60 years). It contains *cytokinins* (plant hormones) which are known for their anti-cancer, anti-ageing and anti-thrombolytic benefits, and is a powerful source of vitamins and minerals, electrolytes, amino-acids, enzymes, phytonutrients and anti-oxidants.

○ A mug of hot water with lemon is a really beneficial way to start your day. Not only is it a source of vitamin C but it is a great cleanser and prepares your system for breakfast. In spite of being told that this is bad practice due to the effect of the lemon on tooth enamel, I happen to think that if it encourages you to drink more water then the benefits to your overall health, and, spectacularly, to your skin, outweigh this one disadvantage. Just make sure you leave at least half an hour before cleaning your teeth afterwards.

○ Try also, adding a good squeeze of fresh lime or lemon juice to cold water to pep it up and make it more interesting. Use a "glass with class" and add a slice of lemon or lime to lift your drink out of the ordinary into the extra-ordinary!

Summary and Conclusion

Well there you have it, you have reached the end of "The Ultimate Guide to Antiaging", so *Congratulations* for taking the first step in what I hope will be not only an enjoyable but a thoroughly enlightening and result-driven journey. ***Even if you only manage to achieve half of what is in this book you will see a vast improvement in the appearance and condition of your skin, and in your energy levels and general vitality***.

This really is the only way to go that makes perfect, logical sense, not only to prevent wrinkles but to massively improve the appearance of existing ones, and to give you radiantly beautiful and supercharged skin from top to toe. All this *without* the need for risky surgeries and procedures, or any astronomical costs, just the right knowledge, some basic lifestyle changes and small amounts of healthy, delicious food!

While there may seem to be an awful lot of information to take in, the basic concept (in a nutshell) is really very simple … eliminate the foods that are known to be bad for you and that have no nutritional value whatsoever, and eat a wide variety of the rest (from all major food groups) in moderation! The same principle applies to all those toxins and chemicals that need eradicating from your life – but if you really are finding it difficult to process all the information, then resolve to make just two healthier substitutions every day, maybe increasing it to three or four after a few weeks or whenever you feel ready to move forward again (I'm really trying to make things easy here!).

To help make certain transitions easier, think at first "*I will try to avoid*" rather than "*I can never have.*" and remember that to make even one change is better than to make no change at all. **One change leads to another as your body noticeably starts to respond to your improved lifestyle choices, and you will both look and feel so much younger than before. You will start to exude that elusive "inner glow", friends and family will begin to comment, and as a result you will feel increasingly confident**.

Try, however, to keep nice and relaxed about things – as realistically you cannot provide yourself with complete immunity from 21st century living, and you need to accept that there will be times when you are not able to follow your new régime as much as you would like (for instance when you are away, or eating out with friends). This is all about making informed and improved lifestyle choices that will benefit you in both the short and the long-term - just don't become too obsessive as it will cause you to be anxious and stressed and may compromise the overall effectiveness of the plan.

Work on those major issues applicable to you that will bring about the quickest and most noticeable changes namely *smoking* and *excessive alcohol consumption*, prolonged and unprotected *sun exposure, insufficient hydration*, dangerously *high levels of sugar, trans fats, refined foods and toxic chemicals* in your diet, *insufficient exercise*, and – most importantly - a *lack of naturally nutritious and healthy foods*. Address these issues and everything else will fall into place.

You will notice a nice and gradual weight loss, decreased stress levels, a better quality sleep and increased energy to deal with everything life throws at you on a day-to-day basis. Most of all you will have Smashed That Clock and called time on ageing skin for good!

Thank you for reading, good luck and above all make your journey fun!

Ps ... If you have enjoyed my book and found it useful, it would be greatly appreciated if you left a review so others can benefit from the same information. Your review will help me see what is and isn't working, or if there is anything that I can do to improve the quality or presentation of any future guides. Many thanks!

Bonus Section 1 - Items you may find useful (and *without* needing to spend much money!)

Blender/Food Processor

For making soups, smoothies etc. This item is probably the most essential.

Bread Making Machine

Fill your house with the heavenly aroma of baking bread.

Slow Cooker

Ideal for one pot meals with meat, fish (or vegetarian alternative) and lots of lovely vegetables.

Steamer

For a healthier way of cooking vegetables.

Juicer

For when you want to extract the juice alone, from fruits and vegetables.

Nutcrackers

For cracking those healthier unshelled nuts, fun for all the family!

Recipe book for bread-making

Recipe books (general)

Look out in particular for Mediterranean cook books where you should find plenty of healthy recipes using chicken, fish and vegetables. Also, on your travels, any recipe collections from farm shops, tea rooms etc., which will be biased towards home cooking with fresh and seasonal produce.

Look for these items in your local charity shops, local bargain pages or on EBay. There is no need to pay full price for anything these days. Cut recipes out of your favourite magazines - I've found some lovely recipes only recently in the free magazines that come with the "Sunday Express" and "The Mail on Sunday". Remember that most recipes can be adapted by the simple substitution of healthy ingredients for unhealthy ones and – if you are vegetarian – by using meat substitutes such as quorn or tofu, in place of meat.

Bonus Section 2 – Natural skincare

This niche area of skincare is massive and would fill a book twice the size of this one! However I have included a very general overview here, as it is something that may well be of interest to some people. Hopefully there will be enough information to provide a springboard for further reading and experimenting to suit your own particular requirements.

When we talk about natural skincare, we are talking about preparations for your skin that you make yourself at home from ingredients you may already have in your store cupboard, and using natural oils, either as a base or, in the case of concentrated essential oils, by adding a couple of drops to the final preparation to add a particular benefit. Basically, once you know what is good for what you can make up your own preparations using organic and unprocessed ingredients which (if you have reached this point in the book) you will now be starting to buy in anyway, for your store cupboard.

You can also search the internet to find literally dozens of different recipes for skincare "from the kitchen table" as it were!

As mentioned earlier in the book, synthetic oils can seriously affect your skin by clogging its pores and causing it to become dry and irritable. To strengthen and tone your skin from within you should be looking at natural skin toning oils for use on your face and body, such as **avocado, jojoba, almond, grape seed** and **coconut**. These are all excellent anti-oxidants, and will protect your skin from ageing and disease whilst they firm and nourish it at a deep level.

Avocado oil is an absolute power-house of anti-oxidants, vitamins, fatty acids and sterolins. It is a highly nutritious and deeply penetrating oil, and has been proven *to actively promote the production of collagen in the skin* to prevent sagging and wrinkles. It can also help in reversing damage caused by the sun and other factors, and is an effective treatment against age spots and scar tissue.

Jojoba oil is another very powerful anti-oxidant which works deep down to prevent the formation of lines, wrinkles and saggy skin. It too, has healing properties due to its natural *vitamin E* content, and it is also a really beautiful and nourishing moisturizer. Because of the fact that its composition is very like the oils secreted by your own skin, it is easily and readily accepted and absorbed by your skin.

Almond oil is one of the best ingredients you can use to reverse the signs of ageing, due in no small part to its high content of *vitamin E*. Additionally it is a rich source of *vitamin D, magnesium, calcium*, and also *oleic acid* which helps to clean, moisturize and lubricate your skin.

Almond oil has been used over many centuries as a treatment for minor cuts and abrasions, and as a soothing balm for dry, inflamed or irritated skin. It is super-nourishing and will smooth, soften and add moisture to any skin type. It is also an excellent remedy for lightening dark circles under the eyes. Simply soak a cotton wool bud and apply gently under the eyes every night to see a significant improvement.

Grapeseed oil also contains high levels of *vitamin E* which ensures powerful healing and anti ageing effects. It is excellent at reducing stretch marks and improving the condition and appearance of unhealthy skin, and its astringent properties make it great for toning and tightening. In addition it is easily penetrable, and is known to play an important role in maintaining levels of collagen and elastin in the skin.

Coconut oil in its purest form is another wonderful anti-ageing moisturizer, a powerful anti-oxidant that is resistant to oxidation and free radical formation. With regular use it keeps your connective tissues strong and supple, and it is a natural exfoliant that will gently smooth the surface of your skin without removing the natural oils that are essential to repair and protect it. Coconut oil is also anti-viral and anti-bacterial. Almost 50% of its fat is healthy *lauric acid* (which, if you use the oil in cooking, converts naturally in your body to *monolaurin*, a substance that inhibits the growth of almost every strain of bacteria).

All these oils are readily available in your local health food stores and from larger branches of Boots, and of course you can purchase them from many online sources.

Concentrated essential oils, which can be added to any skincare recipe to add a particular benefit, include *lavender* and *chamomile* (relaxing and soothing), *peppermint* and *eucalyptus* (astringent and energy boosting) and *ginger* (anti-inflammatory). You will need only two or three drops, as a rule, to reap the full and wonderful benefits of essential oils.

Other natural substances we should be looking at include *organic honey* (preferably manuka*)*, *fruits* (for example pineapple ,bananas, lemons, strawberries, apricots, grapes and tomatoes), *dairy products* (milk, yoghurt and eggs), *aloe vera, sea salt, olive oil*, and of course the vast choice of wonderful *herbs* and *spices* given to us by Mother Nature! I will talk briefly about just a few of these before bringing this section to a close with a small selection of very basic skincare recipes that I hope will give you an idea of the sort of thing you can quite easily do at home.

Honey (in particular manuka honey) is not only a natural skin treat but a luxurious anti-ageing substance. It is a rich source of *minerals*, the *B vitamins* and *vitamin C*, and it has anti-oxidant and anti-inflammatory properties when applied directly to your skin. As honey attracts water, it is an effective moisturiser when applied daily to your face. Apply in a smooth layer and leave for 15-30 minutes before washing off thoroughly.

Aloe vera is an amazing plant with multiple benefits for your skin and general health. It has been used therapeutically for centuries due to its healing and soothing properties stemming from a multitude of active components. These include a rich supply of vitamins and minerals (aloe is one of the few plants to contain vitamin B12), amino acids (the "building blocks" of protein) and fatty acids.

Every part of the aloe plant can be utilized from the oil and the juice to the gel, which is found in the leaf and is 99% water. This high water content means that aloe gel is very hydrating and moisturizing and helps to repair and rejuvenate the skin, improving its appearance and texture by softening the dead skin cells of the epidermis and leaving the skin velvety soft. Its high content of vitamins C and E also helps improve hydration and boost levels of collagen and elastin, thus improving the skin's elasticity. With regular use it can noticeably reduce the visibility of stretch marks.

Aloe is great for sensitive skin as it is non-irritating and immensely soothing. It also contains anti-inflammatory, antiseptic and antimicrobial properties that render it ideal for treating blemishes in acne sufferers, for healing wounds, or for applying topically to burns - and the gel is commonly used to reduce the pain and inflammation of sunburn and to replenish lost moisture to dry, sun burnt skin. And as if all that was not enough, aloe is also antibiotic, antibacterial, antiviral and anti-fungal.

Pineapple is a lovely natural exfoliant due to the particular enzymes it contains. You can either pat the fresh juice directly onto your skin, or combine with natural yoghurt to give a cooling, smoothing and hydrating facial mask with not a chemical in sight!

Strawberries have natural astringent properties and, as with pineapple, the fresh juice can be patted straight onto the skin to tone and firm.

Lemon is also an astringent and is particularly good for oily skin. Pat a few drops of fresh juice on your skin, or add a couple of drops to any skincare recipe to enjoy its brightening and toning effects. Additionally a few drops of fresh lemon massaged into your toenails will keep them looking light and bright. Lemon is also full of vitamins and minerals essential to healthy hair, and is especially beneficial for oily hair or to rid your hair of shampoo build-up: simply dilute the juice of a lemon in some water (about a glassful) and apply it to your hair and scalp, leaving for a few minutes before rinsing well and washing as usual.

Apple cider vinegar, like green tea, is an anti-inflammatory that can help take the sting out of sunburn and insect bites. It is also effective in reducing acne. Simply apply it neat to the skin, leave on for 5-15 minutes and then rinse off. Like lemon juice it has astringent properties that reduce the build-up of oil or shampoo on your hair when diluted with about 3 parts water…leave on your hair for 5 minutes or so then rinse off well.

Olive oil is a great moisturiser that works well as a "mixer" with, for example, sea salt or brown sugar as an exfoliant. Use the best quality, organic oil that you can find for this purpose.

Egg White is great for helping get rid of under-eye bags as it is a rich source of proteins and amino acids. To see results you need do no more than dip your finger in a small amount of egg white and dab under your eyes, then leave for 10-15 minutes.

Ground sea salt makes a good exfoliator when mixed with olive oil, or indeed any massage oil, and rubbed on the face or body with a circular motion. Once you have your basic mix then you can add other ingredients if you wish, for example a couple of drops of your favourite essential oil.

If you have an oily skin type then you could mix the salt in some honey instead. I personally find this all far too harsh and abrasive (if you remember I advised that exfoliation should be carried out with extreme caution) and so would opt to use soft brown sugar instead. However the benefits of sea salt as a healer cannot be underestimated, and a mineral salt bath will do wonders for the health and condition of your skin.

Ground ginger added to any skincare preparation acts as an effective anti-inflammatory which can help with any inflammatory skin condition when used on a regular basis.

Cinnamon is especially good for spotty or pimply skin when mixed with a little honey.

Chamomile is not only a soothing drink but a great toner for your skin. Simply brew up some chamomile, dip a cotton wool ball in the brew and apply it to your face directly, or mix with a little cornflower to make a paste, leaving on your face for 5-10 minutes before rinsing off. Chamomile also has anti-inflammatory properties, so can help heal blemishes and keep wrinkles at bay.

Herbs like chamomile have been used for centuries to prevent disease and promote healing, and they have many and varied uses when it comes to anti-ageing and to reducing your physical and mental decline.

Ginseng, for example, has amazing stress-busting properties, and also very positive effects on your immune system.

Ashwagandha, used in traditional Indian medicine, contains natural anti-oxidants, can reduce anxiety and depression and also strengthen your immune system.

St John's wort, most often used to treat depression and insomnia, can also help the body to repair damage caused by daily stress and oxidation.

Gingko biloba has long been used in traditional Chinese medicine to increase the levels of oxygen in the brain, thus improving memory and cognitive function.

And finally I will give a mention to **Gotu Kola**, a herb that is little known generally but that has remarkable restorative properties both to heal and rejuvenate the skin, restoring its radiant and youthful appearance. Just a word of caution here, as some herbs are so potent that they can have adverse effects on medication you may be taking. I would advise, therefore, that if you are taking prescribed medication you check with your GP before adding any herb to your régime on a regular basis.

Here are some easy "beginner" recipes that you can easily make and try out for yourself to give you an idea of what it's all about. Don't be afraid to experiment and add different ingredients according to your skin type and any particular problems you may have, and of course you are free to create your own unique preparations to your liking.

If this is something that you feel you want to explore further then the internet is awash with websites offering free information and recipes for natural skincare – or browse your local charity shops for books on the subject.

Face Masks for Dry Skin
Use 2-3 times a week depending upon how dry your skin is

- Combine **1 egg yolk**, **2 teaspoons almond oil** and **1 ripe banana** in a bowl to make a thick paste. Apply to your face and neck, leave for 20-30 minutes then rinse off with warm water.
- Mash **½ a ripe avocado** until nice and smooth. Apply to your face, leave for 10-15 minutes then gently remove with a damp cloth.

Face Masks for Oily Skin
Use once a week, but if your skin is very oily use twice a week

- Mix together **1 beaten egg white**, **1 teaspoon honey**, and **1 teaspoon lemon juice** (plus a little of the pulp if liked). Smooth this mask over your face, leave for 10-15 minutes then wash off with warm water.

- Combine **1 tablespoon honey** and **1 tablespoon rose water** with **1 tablespoon Fuller's Earth**. Apply to your skin, leave for 15 minutes then wash off with warm water.

- Mix **1 teaspoon tomato pulp** with **2 tablespoons potato flour** (available in health food stores). Apply to your face, leave for 15 minutes then remove gently with warm water.

You could add extra impact to any of these three masks by adding two to three drops of a naturally astringent essential oil such as eucalyptus.

Face Masks for Normal Skin
Use once a week

- Mix **1 beaten egg white** with **2 teaspoons almond oil**. Smooth over your face and neck, leave for 15 minutes then remove gently with water.

- Blend together **1 egg white**, **2teaspoons olive oil** and **1teaspoon apple juice**. Use as above.

- Mash **1 ripe papaya** and smooth over your face and throat. Leave for 15 minutes, wash off with warm water then splash your face with cold water.

Skin Lightening Remedies
These remedies are useful for restoring an even tone to blotchy or discoloured skin. They are effective in reducing the appearance of freckles and to brighten fading tans, and can also help lighten the appearance of stretch marks.

- Mix some **fresh lemon juice** to a paste with some **finely ground sea salt**. Apply to your skin and leave for ½ hour, then rinse off. Repeat daily. This action may lighten brown patches caused by the sun.

- Combine **3 tablespoons milk** with **1 teaspoon limejuice**, and sponge over skin to remove a fading tan. Use daily.

- Blend **plain yoghurt** with an equal amount of **buttermilk** and apply as a night cream which will also improve the appearance of a fading tan.

- Smooth some **aloe vera gel** over sun-darkened freckles or age spots at least twice a day. You can buy the gel from a store, but it is far better to use gel squeezed from a fresh aloe vera leaf (available at some more niche stores).

- Place a bunch of fresh, washed **watercress** in a small pan with about **200 mls water** (adjust according to size of the bunch!). Cover and bring to the boil, then simmer for 10 minutes. Strain and store in the fridge. Sponge the chilled liquid over your fading tan every morning and evening, allowing to dry before rinsing off with water.

- **Potato Water** is an old Germanic cure for fading tans and summer freckles. Simply sponge onto your skin the water in which potatoes have been cooked.

Herbal Facial Steam

Bring your choice of **any dried herbs** (for example lavender, chamomile, lemongrass, rosemary etc.) to the boil in a large pan of water. Remove from the heat and pour into a large bowl. Place a cloth over your head and steam your face for five minutes. Immediately afterwards, rinse with cold water. This is a great way to deeply cleanse your pores, and to absorb the wonderful benefits of these herbs that are rich in nutrients to nourish and tone your skin. Finish by applying a deeply penetrating and moisturizing oil like avocado or jojoba.

I hope this has interested you enough to want to find out more about natural skincare. As I said earlier there are literally dozens of recipes available on the internet for free that sound so good you could eat them, and all of which will have inestimable benefits for your skin. In the introduction to Section 3, I recommended that you should continue to use a minimal amount of moisturizer on your skin while it is adjusting to its new régime and this the ideal time to experiment with some of the wonderful natural oils and other substances that will nourish and support your skin from the inside-out.

Bonus Section 3

Some favourite food recipes for you to enjoy!

I have included just a few of my favourite recipes below, to give you an idea of the many ways in which you can use these lovely fresh and natural foods in everyday cooking. Not being an expert cook myself, this is not intended to be a cookery lesson. Many of you will probably be far more skilled in the kitchen than I profess to be! However I do love to try out different dishes and to use the best and freshest ingredients possible, so at the very least you may come across some recipes that you like the sound of and haven't tried before.

The recipes are mostly ones that have been jotted down and passed to me by my many "foodie" friends over the years, and I have no idea of their origins, so if I have inadvertently duplicated someone's original recipe it is completely unintentional and I apologize.

I have categorized the recipes simply as "savoury" and" sweet" (which I hope keeps things simple!) otherwise they are in fairly random order. **Remember to use the very best quality food you can afford - preferably organic and, in the case of meat and eggs, free range - and substitute natural and unrefined ingredients for processed and unhealthy ones**.

As I said above, most recipes you come across can be adapted using these simple rules. If organic is not possible for any reason then, in the case of fruit and vegetables, to eat non-organic is better than not to eat them at all but do think carefully about the very real benefits of organic produce.

SAVOURY RECIPES

Watercress and Lime Soup
Serves 6

Ingredients
50g (2oz) *butter*
250g (8oz) diced *potato*
250g (8oz) chopped *leeks*
3 bunches of *watercress*, stalks removed
1¾ pints organic *vegetable stock* (home-made even better!)
Grated rind and juice of 1 *lime*
Seasoning to taste
4 tablespoons *cream*
Watercress sprigs for garnish

Method
1. Melt the butter in a large pan. Gently cook the potato and leeks for 10 minutes
2. Finely chop the watercress
3. Pour the stock into the pan and bring to the boil
4. Add the cress and simmer for 8 minutes. Do not overcook

5. Carefully pour into a blender, in batches if necessary, and purée until smooth
6. Return to the pan, add the lime juice and rind, and seasoning to taste, then heat through
7. Serve with a swirl of cream and a sprig of watercress

Red Pepper and Almond Soup
Serves 4

Ingredients
3 *red peppers* quartered, cored & de-seeded
3 tbs *organic olive oil*
1 *onion*, peeled and chopped
Finely grated rind of ½ a small *orange*
50g (1¾ oz) *ground almonds*
600ml (1pt) organic *vegetable stock*
Sprinkle of *salt* and freshly ground *black pepper*
2 tbsp *crème frâiche* or *single cream*

Method
1. Place the peppers, skin-side uppermost, on a foil-lined grill rack and grill for 15mns or until charred
2. Remove the peppers and place in a plastic bag to cool for about 10mns – after which gently peel away the skins
3. Heat the oil in a pan, then add the onions, almonds and orange rind
4. Stir gently for about 5 mins until the onions have softened and the almonds are starting to colour

5.   Add the peppers and the stock, then simmer gently for about 5mns
6.   Leave to cool, then transfer to a blender and purée until smooth
7.   Return to the pan and heat through, swirling in the crème frâiche or cream
8.   Serve topped with a sprinkle of toasted almonds if liked, and a sprig of fresh basil

Note: this recipe can be adapted for use with fennel rather than peppers. Simply substitute two to three fennel bulbs, trimmed and quartered, then follow the recipe from step 3. Make sure the fennel is completely soft at the end of step 5. You will need to allow a slightly longer cooking time of around 15 minutes.

Pumpkin and Sweet Potato Soup
Serves 6

Ingredients
1kg *pumpkin flesh*
450g *sweet potatoes*
50g *butter*
2 *onions*, sliced
5cm piece of *stem ginger*, peeled & chopped
2 tsps *caraway seeds*
1.7 litres organic *vegetable stock*
2 tsps of clear *organic honey or agave nectar*
½ tbsp *cinnamon*
Pinch of *nutmeg*

Method
1.   Quarter and peel the pumpkin with a sharp, strong knife and cut roughly into cubes
2.   Melt the butter in a large pan and sauté the onions for 5 mins
3.   Add the pumpkin, sweet potato, ginger, caraway seeds, stock and seasoning, then cover and simmer gently for 15-20 mins
4.   Transfer to a blender in batches and purée until smooth, then return to the pan
5.   Add the honey, cinnamon and nutmeg, then bring back to the boil
6.   Serve on its own or with crusty whole-grain bread

Pea and Watercress Salad with melted Goats Cheese

Serves 4

Ingredients
3 tbsp *organic olive oil*
1 tbsp *wholegrain mustard*
2 *oranges*, peeled and segmented, plus 30 ml of juice reserved
200g *goat's cheese* (eg Chevre Blanc)
175g cooked *petit pois* (fresh or frozen)
75g bag of organic *watercress*
Seasoning to taste

Method
1.   Preheat the grill to high

2.   Mix together the mustard, oil, juice and some seasoning then set aside
3.   Slice the cheese into 4 rounds, place on a foil-lined grill pan and grill until bubbling and golden
4.   Allow to cool slightly before removing with a palette knife
5.   Toss the peas, watercress and orange segments with the dressing and divide attractively between four plates
6.   Top each with a round of the grilled goat's cheese and some fresh ground black pepper

Creamy Scrambled Eggs with Asparagus
Serves 2

Ingredients
4 large free-range *eggs*, lightly beaten
½ oz *butter*
½ tbsp *olive oil*
70 ml *single cream*
1 bunch fresh *asparagus*
Freshly chopped *chives* to garnish
Seasoning to taste

Method
1.   Preheat a grill pan
2.   Wash and trim the asparagus then lightly coat in olive oil and season with a little salt and freshly ground black pepper

3. Line the grill pan with a piece of foil and place the asparagus on it
4. Grill in a single layer, turning frequently, until the asparagus is very slightly charred on all sides
5. Melt the butter in a small pan, then add the beaten eggs and cream
6. Cook very gently, stirring and folding the eggs with a spatula until they are soft and creamy
7. Serve on a bed of asparagus and garnish with a few chives

Cheesy Stuffed Mushrooms

Serves 4

This delicious recipe is so, so quick and easy to make ... if you're not confident with cooking then try this to start with, it's virtually foolproof!

Ingredients

4 large flat *mushrooms*
1 cup grated *mature cheddar cheese*
½ cup *onions*, finely grated
3 tbsp *mayonnaise*
1 level tsp *curry powder* or *cumin* (add more to taste, if liked)
Fresh ground *black pepper*

Method

1. Remove the stalks of the mushrooms and place upside down on a baking tray
2. Mix all the rest of the ingredients, binding together with the mayo and use this mixture to stuff the mushrooms

3.   Put in a pre-heated oven 200ºc/Gas Mark 6 for 10 minutes
4.   Transfer under the grill for 3-4 minutes until brown and bubbling
5.   Serve with a fresh green salad

Note: you can also make this dish using halved peppers instead of mushrooms

Prawns Pil Pil - aka Garlic Prawns
Serves 2 as a starter or tapas dish

Ingredients
300g uncooked *prawns*
2tbsp *olive oil*
4 *garlic* cloves, chopped
pinch of *paprika*
pinch of **salt**
2tbsp *dry sherry* (optional)

Method
1.   Pour the oil into a small pan and heat until simmering
2.   Add the chopped garlic and paprika and heat gently, stirring. Do not let the garlic turn brown
3.   Add the prawns, sherry (if using) and seasoning, then cook until the prawns change colour.
4.   Serve with crusty wholewheat bread to mop up the delicious juices

Avocado and Prawn Cocktail
Serves 2

Ingredients
1 *very ripe avocado*, halved and stoned
150g cooked and peeled *prawns*
4 tbsp *mayonnaise*
small piece of *root ginger*, grated (enough for 1 tsp)
1 tbsp organic *passata* (if you have no passata then just use tomato ketchup)
1 *lime*, half juiced and half cut into wedges
freshly ground *black pepper*

Method
1.   Scoop the flesh out of each avocado half
2.   Stir the root ginger and passata into the mayonnaise and mix together
3.   Chop the avocado flesh and mix with the prawns, lime juice and ginger mayonnaise
4.   Fill the avocado shells with the mixture, season with black pepper and serve garnished with a wedge of lime

Home-made Ratatouille
A colourful side dish packed with nutrition

Ingredients
1 *aubergine*
1 *red pepper*
1 *yellow pepper*

Rosi Thomas

1 *fennel bulb*
1 *courgette*
2 cloves of *garlic* (add more to taste)
1 *red onion*
2 large *beef tomatoes*
fresh *oregano* and *thyme* to taste
organic olive oil

You can adapt the amounts of each vegetable to suit your taste, but the above is a guide as to what you might use. If you wish you can use a tin of chopped tomatoes in place of the beef tomatoes, but as always fresh is best!

Method
1.   Cut up all the above ingredients into very small "dice-like" pieces (although this can be a time-consuming exercise, try not to prepare your vegetables more than an hour in advance as you will lose valuable nutrients.)
2.   Pour about a tbsp of olive oil into a large pan, cook the onions until almost soft then add the garlic and cook for another 2-3 minutes
3.   Add the rest of the ingredients (add a little more oil if necessary) with a sprinkle of salt and black pepper to taste, then cook slowly for 30-40 minutes
4.   Finely chop the herbs and add to the mixture about half way through the cooking time

Mediterranean Salad with Croutons
Serves 6

Ingredients

6 large, ripe and fragrant *vine tomatoes*, roughly chopped

1 red, green or yellow *pepper*, cored and sliced

1 *red onion*, thinly sliced

1 *garlic* clove, finely sliced

2 tbsp small *capers*, drained

150g/5oz pitted *black olives* (or olives of your choice)

8 tbsp *extra virgin olive oil*

2 tbsp *red wine vinegar*

1 small bunch fresh *basil*

1 small *ciabatta* type loaf

Method

1. Combine the tomatoes, pepper, onion, garlic, olives and capers in a large serving dish

2. Whisk the oil and vinegar together and stir into the salad

3. Season with a little ground sea salt and some black pepper

4. Split the ciabatta and grill on a ridged pan until just charred at the edges

5. Break into small croutons, mix in well with the salad and scatter over some torn basil leaves

Enjoy with a little strong cheese and a glass of wine, perfect for a summer evening!

Whipped Stilton with pear and watercress

Serves 4

Ingredients
225g/8oz *stilton*
2 *pears,* quartered then halved again
1 heaped tbsp chopped *walnuts*
1 bunch *watercress*, washed & torn into sprigs
125-150ml *crème frâiche*
Crushed *sea salt* and ground *black pepper*

For the Dressing
1 tbsp *redcurrant jelly*
1 tbsp *red wine vinegar*
1 tbsp *port*
4 tbsp *walnut or olive oil*
Sea salt and ground *black pepper*

Method
1.   Crumble the Stilton into a small food processor and blend until soft and creamy. To achieve this consistency add 125-150ml of crème frâiche according to taste. Keep at room temperature for a soft consistency, or chill for a firmer finish
2.   Whisk together the redcurrant jelly, port and red wine vinegar in a bowl until smooth, then stir in the oil and season with salt and pepper to taste
3.   Divide the stilton mix between 4 plates, in an attractive swirl
4.   Arrange the pear pieces alongside the stilton, topped with watercress sprigs and chopped walnuts
5.   Drizzle with redcurrant dressing and a smidge of seasoning

Note: if you wish, fresh *figs* can be substituted for pears (about 6, quartered) which works equally well. And if you want to make the dish more substantial then add a slice of *walnut bread* to accompany it.

Spanish Almonds

A tasty and delicious way to eat these nutritious nuts!

Ingredients

200g/7oz *blanched almonds*
25g/1oz *butter*
4 tbsp *olive oil*
2 tbsp best quality, unrefined *sea salt*
¼ tsp *cayenne pepper*

Method

1. Stir together the salt and cayenne pepper in a bowl
2. Melt the oil and butter in a large but shallow pan
3. Fry the almonds, stirring, until golden brown. Do not allow them to burn and become blackened
4. Transfer the almonds carefully from the pan into the salt mixture and coat evenly
5. Leave to cool before storing in an airtight container for about a week

Sweet Potato Cakes with Oats

Serves 4

Rosi Thomas

Ingredients
400g *sweet potatoes*
small knob of *butter*
2oz mature *cheddar cheese*, grated
4 small *spring onions*, chopped
1 tsp *organic vegetable stock powder*
2 tsps *wholegrain mustard*
40g *oats*
a little crushed *sea salt* and freshly ground *black pepper*

Method
1.   Peel the potatoes and cut into wedges, then boil gently until soft
2.   Drain and mash with a tiny bit of butter, just enough to help them mash easily, too much liquid and they will be difficult to handle
3.   Add the chopped onions, the cheese, the mustard and the stock powder
4.   Form into 8 balls, flatten out into "cakes" and roll in the oats seasoned with salt and pepper to taste
5.   Dry fry in a non-stick pan brushed lightly with oil, 3-4 minutes each side or until crisp and golden
6.   Serve with a green or mixed salad or some left-over ratatouille from the day before!

I sometimes adapt this recipe by replacing the *grated cheese, stock powder and mustard* from Step 3 with *150g (50z) salmon fillet*, poached and roughly flaked, the *finely grated zest of an orange*, a clove or two of *chopped garlic* and a small bunch of *shredded parsley*. The method otherwise remains the same.

Baked salmon with tomatoes and fennel
Serves 6

Ingredients
1 large *fennel bulb*, trimmed and cut into wedges
3 large sticks of *celery* cut into approx. 3inch pieces
700g (1½ lbs) *salmon fillet*, divided into 6 chunks
6 lovely ripe *plum* or *vine tomatoes*, halved
1 large *onion,* sliced
handful fresh *dill*, chopped
5 tbsp *vermouth*
1 tbsp *olive oil*
seasoning to taste

Method
1. Preheat the oven to 200°c/Fan 180°c/Gas Mark 6
2. Mix the fennel, celery and onion with the oil and roast on a large tray for 20 mins
3. Turn the vegetables and add the salmon and tomatoes, seasoning with sea salt and freshly ground black pepper
4. Return to the oven for 10 mins
5. Drizzle the vermouth evenly over the dish, and scatter with chopped dill
6. Bake for a further 10 mins until the salmon is cooked through and the vegetables fork tender
7. Serve with hot, fresh-baked bread

Hot and Fruity Tuna
Serves 4

Ingredients
4 *tuna steaks*
3-4 tbsp *olive oil*
teriyaki and *soy sauce* for a marinade
juice of 1 *lemon*
juice of 1 *grapefruit*
1 piece of *stem ginger*, peeled and grated
chopped *coriander* (about 1 tbsp)
freshly ground *black pepper*
1 small *pineapple*, peeled and chopped
1 small *mango*, peeled and chopped
1 small *red pepper*
1 red *chilli pepper*, chopped (or a tsp of *cayenne pepper* if preferred)
½ *red onion*, peeled and sliced

Method
1. Place the tuna steaks in a large dish and completely cover with 50% teriyaki and 50% soy sauces. Put in the fridge *overnight* to marinate
2. Reduce the fresh lemon and grapefruit juice to a syrup over a medium heat
3. Add the grated ginger, pepper and coriander
4. Mix the olive oil with the syrup and allow to stand for 1 hour
5. Meanwhile chop or slice the red pepper, chilli pepper, pineapple, mango and onion
6. Quick fry in a little oil, not letting get too soft
7. Add the syrup to the fruit and mix together

8.	Remove the tuna from the marinade and pat dry
9.	Quick-fry for 4 mins each side, turning once only
10.	Slice each steak into small pieces and serve, hot or cold, with the fruit garnish

Chicken Goulash
Serves 4

This recipe is for a standard size slow cooker. If you prefer, for the chicken, substitute around 700gm (1lb 6oz) of lean, diced pork

Ingredients
8 boneless, skinless *chicken thighs* (or if you prefer, 4 skinless *chicken breasts*, cut into chunks)
1 tbsp *olive oil*
1 large *onion*, chopped
1 *carrot*, cut into chunks
150g (50z) *button mushrooms*, halved
1 tbsp *paprika*, plus extra for garnish (combine with some chilli powder if a hotter dish preferred)
1 tsp *caraway seeds*
½ tsp ground *cinnamon or allspice*
2 tbsp *spelt, buckwheat or wholegrain flour*
400g very ripe *vine or plum tomatoes*, chopped, plus 1tbsp of *tomato purée* or *passata* (you could use a tin of tomatoes here if preferred)
150mls *white wine*
300 mls *organic vegetable stock* (if you make your own so much the better)
seasoning
soured cream and some sprigs of *parsley* for garnish

Method
1.   Preheat the slow cooker
2.   Heat the oil in a pan, then gently cook the chicken, in batches if necessary, over a medium heat until brown on all sides. Remove from the pan with a slotted spoon and keep warm
3.   Add a little more oil to the pan if necessary, then add the onion and sauté until softened
4.   Add the mushrooms and cook gently for a couple more minutes, stirring
5.   Stir in the flour and the spices and cook for a further minute
6.   Add the tomatoes and tomato purée (or canned tomatoes if using) and mix gently
7.   Bring the mixture to the boil then transfer to the slow cooker along with the carrot
8.   Stir in the wine and the stock and season with a little salt and black pepper, then replace the lid and cook on low for 8-10 hours
9.   Garnish with a sprinkle of paprika, a swirl of sour cream and a sprig of parsley, and serve simply with new potatoes and a green vegetable

Note: a slow cooker is a wonderful way to prepare almost any kind of family meal with meat and vegetables. Simply follow the basic principle of the recipe above with your choice of meat, vegetables and seasonings. Root vegetables can be chopped and put in the bottom of the cooker without any pre-cooking required.

Remember that, with ingredients like mushrooms, if you want them to really integrate into the stew and impart the full extent of their flavour, then add them early on in the cooking, but if you would prefer that they held their form and texture then pop them in half- to one hour before the end.

SWEET RECIPES

Fresh Fruit Salad

One of the simplest and most delicious ways to enjoy a variety of your chosen fruits in combination, is to make a lovely bowl of **fresh fruit salad** in natural juice, or for a more adult version add a splash of white wine or a couple of tablespoons of brandy or rum. You should not add extra sugar.

Method
1.   Use as many different coloured fruits as you can - whole, sliced or chopped dependent on the fruit - so that the visual impact is attractively tempting and the dish is crammed with as many different nutrients as possible.   For example you could include a mix of strawberries, kiwi fruit, raspberries, blueberries, melon, and banana
2.   Add juice (enough to just cover) and brandy/rum if using

3. Serve slightly chilled with natural yoghurt or a little single cream, or add a small amount daily to cereal or porridge
4. One large dish will last, and retain its nutritional value, for 5-6 days if kept chilled

Note: fruit is best eaten on an empty stomach rather than after a meal, as it digests so much better.

The next two dishes I **do** know the source of. They are from The Autumn Fruits Cookbook by Charlotte Popescu. I wholeheartedly recommend this book as it is full of delicious, healthy and inexpensive recipes using autumn fruits. You might also like to try another book by the same author called "Vegetables: Grow them, Cook them, Eat them". Incidentally I do not receive any commission from recommending these books; they are just two of my own personal favourites and are well worth investing in. I think I purchased my own copy from a farm shop (price £5.99) but they are also available from several online sources.

Pear and Kiwi Fruit Crunch
A delicious, nutritious and fruity pudding for both children and adults.

Ingredients
3 ripe *pears*, peeled, cored and sliced
juice of ½ *lemon*
3 *kiwi fruits*, peeled and sliced

50g (2oz) *butter*
100g (4oz) wholewheat *breadcrumbs*
50g (2oz) *brown sugar* (I use Billingtons Molasses, a natural unrefined sugar, in this recipe, and actually use a little less than recommended)
1 small tub of *crème frâiche or natural yoghurt*

Method
1. Layer the pears at the bottom of a serving bowl
2. Sprinkle with lemon juice and cover with the sliced kiwi fruit
3. Melt the butter in a small pan and fry the breadcrumbs with the sugar until crisp
4. Spread over the fruit
5. Cover with a layer of crème frâiche or yoghurt
6. I also often sprinkle a few chopped nuts on top, whatever I happen to have in the store-cupboard!

Wheaty Apple and Orange Pudding

Ingredients
3 tbsp *wheatgerm* soaked for 1 hour in the juice of 2 oranges
2 *oranges*
300ml (1/2 pint) *apple purée*
4 tbsp chopped *walnuts*
2 tbsp chopped *almonds*
1 *orange* cut into segments
Grated *rind of 1 orange*
150ml (1/4 pint) *Greek yoghurt*

2 tbsp soft *brown sugar* for sprinkling (again I would use a small amount of Billingtons molasses or similar, or simply decorate with a few extra *chopped nuts* or some *berries*)

Method
1.   Put the soaked wheatgerm into a large serving bowl
2.   Mix the apple purée, walnuts, almonds, orange segments and rind into the wheatgerm
3.   Chill before serving
4.   Spoon over the yoghurt and sprinkle over the sugar, chopped nuts or berries

Valencia Orange and Almond Cake

Ingredients
100g *almonds* (ground) plus a few reserved for decoration
4 medium *free-range eggs*, separated
2 large *oranges*, grated and juiced
1 tbsp *orange liqueur*
150g/5oz **unrefined** *golden castor sugar*
such as Billingtons (I sometimes also use "Total Sweet" as a substitute, with good results)

Method
1.   Preheat the oven to 425ºF/Gas Mark 7
2.   Grease a 26cm cake tin and lightly dust with flour

3. Grind the almonds in a food processor for 2-3 minutes
4. Grate the rind from the oranges
5. Beat the egg yolks with the grated rind and 100g of the sugar until you have a thick creamy mixture
6. Beat in the almonds
7. Whisk the egg whites until stiff and fold into the mixture
8. Spoon into the cake tin and bake for 15mns, then reduce the heat to 330ºF/Gas Mark 3 and bake for a further 15 minutes
9. Cool slightly before removing carefully from the tin and transferring to a flat serving plate
10. Pour the fresh juice from the oranges into a small pan, add the rest of the sugar and stir over a low heat until dissolved
11. Add the orange liqueur then pour the liquid slowly over the cake
12. Sprinkle a handful of extra almonds over the top to decorate
13. Leave overnight for the liquid to soak in and permeate the whole cake with its wonderful flavour

ENJOY!

Printed in Great Britain
by Amazon